Willing to Change

by Kathleen A. Stommel

$W_t C$

Nashville, TN
2005

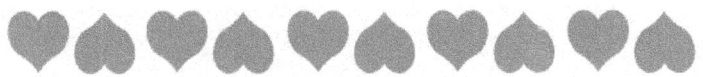

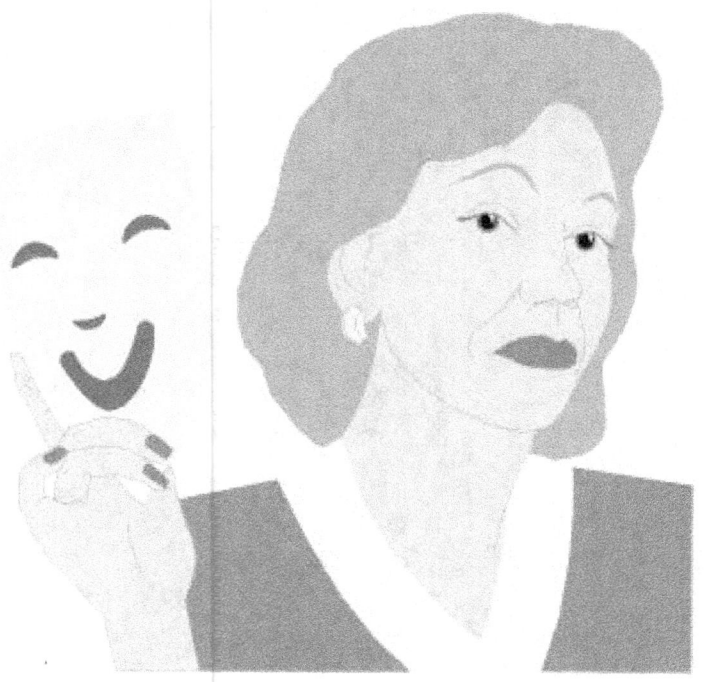

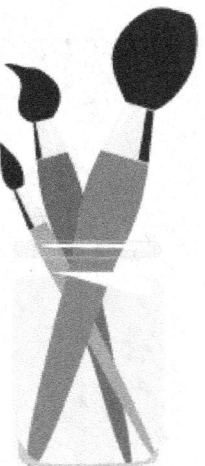

Note to the reader:

It is advisable to seek the guidance of a qualified
health professional before implementing the
planary and other suggestions for specific condi-
tions presented in this book. It is essential that
any reader who has any reason to suspect
serious illness in himself or his family
members seeks appropriate advice. Neither this
nor any other book should be used as a
substitute for qualified care or treatment.

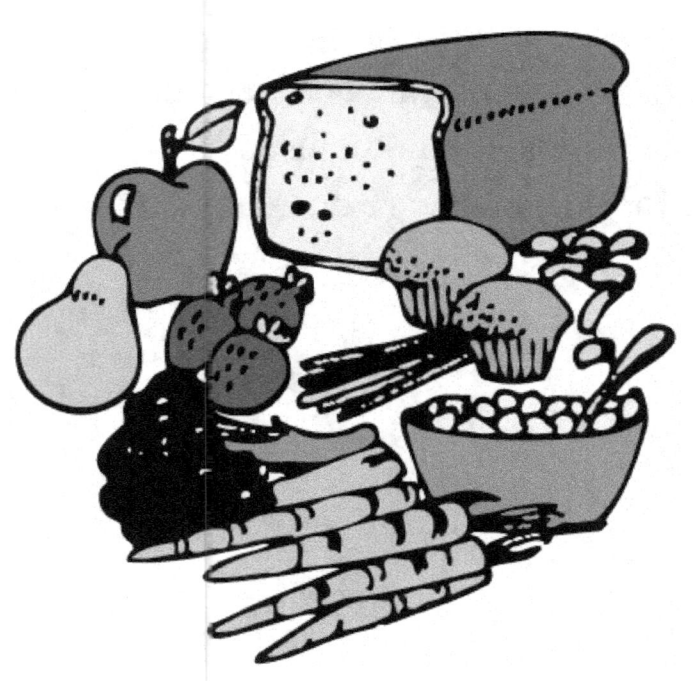

Table of Contents

Table of Contents continued...

Willing To Change

Lose weight and stay your perfect size

-A healthy way of eating, in its most basic form, that sets you free from all plans and obsession with food and weight~

The goal of this book is to help you relearn how to eat in the most simplistic, healthy way so that your body will come back into perfect balance and be at its perfect weight. Our choice of how we eat can merely fill us up and comfort us, or it can heal and transform us.

In two weeks, you will lose weight rapidly .

The Willing To Change Plan starts with a two-week detox program. The plan consists of a foundational, simple food meal plan that is designed to break addictions and attachments to foods that are keeping you fat and slow. When you stick very closely to the foundational two-week meal plan, the body will clean out all unnecessary toxins that keep the body from functioning at its most efficient level. When these toxins are released out of the body, the body can easily do what is needed to lose weight effectively and efficiently and come into a state of health and well-being.

After the two weeks, you can begin Willing to Change-Level II. It has been researched that it takes thirty days, or four weeks, for people to change a habit. The Willing to Change Plan Program is a commitment to four weeks of eating this very simplistic, healthy plan. This is a way to success, starting at one goal of commitment, and then creating a new goal once this goal is achieved. After completing the four-week program, you will have the experience of how it feels to eat healthy and have the benefits of higher levels of energy and well-being. Now it will be easy to continue eating in this way because there will be a desire to do so.

Level II will add more variations of good, healthy food with more calories that are a little bit harder to digest. (Easy digestion makes the body more efficient, resulting in a higher ability to burn calories and fat). The more weight you want to lose, the more you will want to stick with the first two-week plan. Once you have come to your perfect weight goal, you can begin to add more and more variation to your foundational Willing To Change Plan.

What is your desired weight?

Can you see yourself at this desired weight?

Before we start it is very important to get a picture in your mind of how you would like to look and what you would like to accomplish. If you think high (as far as your expectations go), aim high, you will go high and succeed. Before anything is created in this world, it is first imagined in one's mind. Someone "saw" the idea of an umbrella before it was ever created. In order for you to change your body and plan, you must see yourself at your desired weight. You must see yourself able to eat in a new way for a short amount of time…twenty-eight to thirty days (four weeks). Again, this is how long it takes to implement a new habit.

Can you see yourself making a goal and sticking to it?

Every area of your life will benefit just from succeeding at completing a goal. Self-discipline is a powerful force. It strengthens the will. When we strengthen the will, we strengthen our ability to make the dreams in our hearts a reality. This all begins in the mind. If you can't imagine it, it won't happen. When one says, "I can't imagine myself doing that," he will never do what he says he cannot imagine because he has not made it a possibility in his mind. Therefore, he does not have what it takes to bring it to pass.

When you begin to imagine yourself thin, toned, healthy, and eating in a very balanced healthy way without any problems attached to food or body weight, your body begins to cooperate. Your will begins to become engaged. Your mind starts to line up and create solutions to the desired goal. It becomes easier to carry out the tasks that are needed to reach your goal. This step is the beginning foundation that the rest of you will follow.

A Strong 'Will' Brings Success

Your will began developing with your desire to be different in this area of eating and body weight. Your will is strengthened every time you see yourself free of your old ways of eating. Each time you actually eat in a more balanced and healthy way, your will is strengthened even more. A new habit is established, and you become closer and closer to your deliverance from food addictions. I highly recommend finding a picture of yourself at your desired weight. If you do not have one, find a picture in a magazine of a body you would like to be like in size and cut your face out of a picture and put it on top. If this is not desirable, just cover up the face and put it on the refrigerator.

Speak Positively About Yourself

It is also important to begin to tell yourself that you have a thin, toned, healthy, young looking and feeling, beautiful, or great body.

A lot of the time people who are overweight, or who are thinking too much about food, have a lot of dislike for themselves and the way they look. This just creates more defeat when you are trying to change for the better. It is crucial that you start to see and speak about yourself, inside and out, in a more positive way.

Here are some suggestions of positive thoughts and words to replace old, negative thought patterns.

*Everything I eat turns to health and beauty and brings me to my desired weight of _____.
*I like myself.
*I am taking good care of myself by eating a good healthy plan.
*I know how to prepare and buy high quality healthy food.
*I exercise regularly and enjoy it greatly.
*I have a strong will and exercise self control at all times with my eating.
*I am a healthy person.
*I have wisdom when it comes to what to eat, how much, and when to eat it.
*I have all the energy and inspiration I need to prepare, cook and buy good food for myself.
*I've set a goal to eat healthy and exercise daily for four weeks and I'm sticking to it.
*I have what it takes to eat healthy and exercise daily for four weeks.
*I am a thin, toned, energized, healthy individual, and I am free from the bondage of food.

Make a commitment to yourself in writing and hang it up on your bedroom mirror.

I _(*your name*)_____ commit to eating healthy and following the Willing To Change Plan for four weeks. I commit to discipline my body to eat three healthy meals with two healthy snacks, and I will exercise five (or six) times a week. I will stick to this plan no matter what. I have what it takes to stay committed and disciplined. **I am willing to change** .

Sincerely,

_____

Read this every morning and evening.

Why Balanced Eating Works

The **Willing To Change Plan** is a lifestyle of balanced healthy eating. Most people are very confused as to what they are supposed to eat. There is so much information out there on plan and eating. So many reports come out on different foods and supplements that are either good or bad for you. Most of them contradict each other. A lot of them change positions on what they originally stated. I think most people are so confused as to what they should eat, they figure why bother! They are the people who try everything, and their bodies are so confused as to what they are getting next that their body chemistry is never able to come into balance.

When you go on a plan, your body adjusts to that way of eating. Because we are created to survive and thrive on what we feed ourselves, when you stop that particular plan and eat everything you shouldn't have, once again the body has to adjust. It is hard for the body to come into balance when it is going from one extreme to another. Your hormones and body chemicals (that are created to keep your body systems functioning correctly) need a consistent intake of good quality food in order to maintain the proper function to support strength building and healing in your body.

For instance, when we eat a high quantity of sugar, insulin is secreted into the blood stream by the pancreas. Then the liver (which is a filter for the body) has to bring the insulin to its proper level so there is not too much in the blood stream. (When diabetics have too much, they go into what is called diabetic shock; the body has been overloaded with too much of one thing).

The liver and the pancreas then together go to work to bring your blood chemistry into right levels of sugar.

Caffeine

Caffeine from coffee, chocolate, or soft drinks has to be processed by the kidneys. Adrenalin is released from the kidneys into the blood stream and also processed by the liver. (Adrenalin is the same substance that is released by the kidneys when you are afraid. This is that rush you feel if someone comes up behind you and scares you. If you pay attention to how you feel a few minutes later, you will notice that you feel tired and shaky. This is because the body goes to work very hard to process this surge of chemicals. This gives you the ability to have an extra boost of energy to run fast in a dangerous situation. It is an instinctual response from the body to aid survival.) This is what also happens when you are eating high quantities of processed food with additives, dyes, and chemicals, not to mention the consumption of alcohol and over the counter drugs, which are very hard on the liver. The liver has a lot of work to do to detoxify these chemicals out of the body. If it can't get the toxins out right away (because more are coming in), it will store them as fat in the liver, waste in the colon, or fat on the body.

The body is designed to always be in a constant state of cleansing and healing. Whatever you put into your body will begin to break down through digestion into a usable source. The body will throw out all that is not needed or whatever is threatening to the health of your body. If you are constantly putting lots of highly processed, hard to digest food into your system, it will begin to store it until it has a chance to clean it out. There is no time to clean if there is never a break in the intake of toxic foods. This is why a lot of times people become sick after years of eating and drinking poorly. Their bodies become so toxic, imbalances are created, and the body has lost its ability to clean and rejuvenate. Unless the body is given another opportunity to receive a consistent plan of healthy food for a reasonable period of time, the body becomes overloaded and loses its ability to clean and rejuvenate.

Eating poorly will also affect your moods and emotions because of chemical and hormonal imbalances. If the brain does not get the right kind of vitamins and minerals, it doesn't function correctly. When there are hormonal imbalances, you are more tired, fatigued, irritable and cloudy in your thinking. You have too much of one thing and not enough of another. The liver is so over-loaded with toxic chemicals; it cannot maintain proper levels of hormones, sugars, salts, and fats in the body system. So you simply do not think straight. You are under the influence of toxic chemicals in your blood stream.

The amazing thing about the body is that once you take away these toxic foods (even for a short period of time), your body begins to clean out the liver, the colon, then the rest of your body, and begins to build itself back up. We actually grow a new liver every seven years. Our bodies are constantly healing and rejuvenating. Just a cut on your finger will prove that. Within a few days it is healed, and in a week, it will probably be no longer visible. This is the same with every system of the human body.

The Body Like A House

Let's look at it this way; say a man was building a house. The frame was up with walls and a roof. The building materials began to arrive. The men who brought the materials began to bring all kinds of extra supplies. They just kept coming, more and more. The guy building the house said, "Stop! That's enough! It's all I need!" But the men just kept coming. This man could not work. All he could do was work at finding a place to store it all. He could not build until all this "stuff" was out of his way.

This is the same with our bodies. When you keep giving it things that are high in sugar, fat, white flour, etc., all it can do is pull what good it can from it (if there is any good), push out the waste, and store what it cannot process in the form of fat. Eventually, the body is so overloaded it creates cysts or tumors to isolate these chemicals to actually protect the body from these high concentrations of foreign substances.

When you stop taking in highly processed food and start giving the body food that is full of vitamins, minerals and enzymes, the body will immediately be able to easily digest the high quality food and use the nutrients and vitamins to begin the cleansing and healing process. After receiving several meals of high quality food on a consistent basis, the body will now have time to process and assimilate all of the fat and toxic storage in the liver and in other areas of the body.

With the Willing To Change Plan, cleansing is able to take place in a very comfortable way. Many people fast (do not eat for a period of time) to rid their bodies of toxins (which I will discuss later).

But with The Willing To Change Plan, the food
is healthy and clean; it is as if you were on a
fast without having any of the uncomfortable
side effects. (Sometimes fasting can bring toxins
out of the system too quickly for someone who has
been eating poorly for a long time.) This simplistic plan
of healthy eating will bring cleansing, healing and the
desired weight loss . The body can then
take care of any illnesses or problems that have
developed and begin to heal them if
you remains consistent to healthy eating.

How the body works to clean house

The liver is the first organ that the body
begins to work at cleaning out. The colon will
begin to release stored toxins and clogged waste.
(Sometimes this can be experienced as irritabili-
ty or headaches in the early stages of this plan.
This can be slowed down and remedied by eating
a piece of whole grain bread. If it is still very
hard to deal with, a piece of cheese will slow it
down even more…Because cheese is very hard to
digest, the body will go to work on that and temporarily
leave the cleansing process of pulling toxins out
of the body). Once these toxins get out of the
body, you will have much more energy and an
over all good feeling of health and well being.
There are many people who have serious digestive problems as a result of toxic and overloaded
livers, combined with a colon impacted with food
waste that has been stuck for years in their system. The body cannot function the way that it
was created to because of a clogged system.

"This is not difficult!"

Eating this way is very attainable and once practiced, becomes very easy and satisfying. I think we all have become too accustomed to how we've been taught to eat. We derive too much comfort from habits and patterns of eating, often times out of sentimental reasons, because this is what brought us comfort, stability and structure in the past. We are such creatures of habit, and change can bring a sense of vulnerability. But once we commit to a new way of eating, for a certain amount of time, this new way of eating will become the more comfortable choice. The revelation will be in place. This way of eating brings too many benefits to ignore. I think the best benefit of all is the freedom to eat what you want on occasion, knowing if you come back to this foundational plan, indulging will not put weight on you. The "not so good" food will be out of your system efficiently, and with very little side effects.

The Changes

The specific changes that you will have to alter are in the way you grocery shop, and the way you prepare and cook your food. Once you get the hang of it, it is very easy. The standard American plan may seem easier because it is familiar, but the expense, time, and planning all work out to be equal. I have tried both.

I also reason that when you do eat a lot of fast foods, precooked frozen foods, and are not getting the nutrients you need, the effects of this on your body actually slow you down so much that you are losing time because you can't get as much done in this more sluggish state. The

American standard plan is NOT good for you! Packaged, processed, white flour, sugary, fat filled foods will make you fat, depressed, oppressed, slow and cloudy thinking. And eventually, you will get sick if you are excessive in eating these foods. A balanced plan of grains, vegetables, fruit, beans and occasional lean meats will bring vitality, health, and a high quality of life.

This is not difficult, just different. This is why we call this way of eating, "Willing To Change" because that is the whole idea in a nutshell. Are you willing to change? You do not have to do a lot of excessively hard things, but just simply change your eating habits. And this requires the courage to do it differently than Mama and Aunt MeMe. And sometimes this can rattle our cages. But, if you look at it as an opportunity to grow in potential as an independent, free, courageous individual, then this could be a springboard to strengthen you and propel you forward toward the dreams of your heart, which is all about courage and change, also. Once we know we can attain a goal that has been a challenge and hurdle in the past, we become more confident in our ability to do this again and again. Each time we take on something we never thought we could do before and master it, we are stronger for it. If you set your mind and will to say, "I am going to do this. I can do this. This is easy". Your emotions and actions *will* follow.

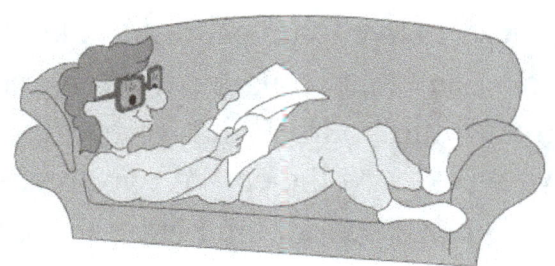

Willing to Change

Getting Started

This is the beginning foundational plan. For two weeks we will be limiting certain foods in order to break cycles of addictions both physically and emotionally. These are the most important foods that we want to stay away from: sugar, white flour, dairy, caffeine, and meat (only for two weeks). These are the most addictive and most clogging substances to our systems. They keep the body working very hard. Once you begin, you will notice a dramatic change in how you feel. You will lose weight in these two weeks.

These two weeks will be a cleansing time for the body. It is important to drink a lot of water, as toxins will be clearing out of your system. These two weeks are the hardest part of eating to lose weight and keep it off. These two weeks are what help you to lose weight quickly and break off cravings that have been hard to control.

It is important to come into these two weeks gradually. Take three days to a week if you have to, to start cutting back on coffee, sweets, cheese, breads and meats. Each day eat less of each food group and gradually cut one out at a time. This will ease any withdrawal symptoms. (For example, if you drink two cups of coffee a day, have one and a half the next day, then one the day after that, then a half a cup the following day, etc. If you eat a lot of meat, start cutting down and then moving to chicken or fish instead of red meat.) If you start having bad headaches, pull out a little more slowly. This doesn't have to be painful. Take it slow and easy.

Pick a day that you are definitely going to start. Commit within yourself that you will stick to this plan for two weeks. At the end of two weeks, you will feel so good. You will be looking better, thinking clearer and having more energy, and you will be able to start adding more variety to your plan. This decision will raise the quality of your life.

As you enter the two weeks of cleansing, you may start to experience some uncomfortable symptoms of withdrawal. It is very important that you stay committed and disciplined, as the outcome far outweighs any passing discomfort. Each day you will feel better and better. Sometimes it's just a matter of hours, and it will pass. Drinking more water, vegetable juices, and sometimes, if it's just too much to bear, eating a piece of whole grain bread will slow down the cleansing effects of withdrawal. Remember that the suffering is breaking food's power over you. This strengthening of the will is what you need to be a life long healthy eater.

Willing To Change Eating Plan

The proportions suggested in each meal can be varied to a *lesser* degree. The most important revelation you can have about how much you eat is to listen to the body's signals while eating. For example, if you are eating nuts, usually by the eighth or ninth nut, the nuts become pasty tasting, (where at first they were very flavorful with many subtle hints of sweet, salty, and the flavor of the nut…almond, peanut, etc). This is the body letting you know that it has had enough. Most of us keep eating after the best taste has gone out of the food, usually out of habit or boredom. This is what leads to excessive fat on the body. In order to reverse this process, you must become very conscious of your eating during the eating process. This is true of all food. After eating a certain amount of food, it will not taste as good as when you first started eating. This is the time to put down the fork or spoon and stop eating. You will do yourself a tremendous favor.

Ninety percent of all weight loss success is the cutting back on your food consumption. This is why *any* plan will bring weight loss when followed correctly. Every plan dictates a certain amount of food a day. It doesn't matter if you are eating frozen dinners, protein drinks, eating all protein, or no sweet vegetables or fruit, eating special bars, etc. The bottom line is that there is a restriction on the amount of food you eat a day. If there isn't, the food is probably some very low calorie drink, fruit, or vegetable that won't give you more calories than you need.

If you can get a handle on how much you eat at a time, and overall in one day, you will never again have to deal with being overweight. The key is to always make food choices that will have a good effect on your health, and *in moderation* have the treats you desire…always returning to healthy food as your foundational plan. Eating just frozen or pre-made meals, eating only protein, or bars and shakes will eventually deprive your body of much needed whole foods. Whole foods are healing as well as natural weight regulators and bring vitality to all the cells of your body. Remember, it's the cutting back of food combined with exercise that brings weight loss. But when you do eat whole foods, you will speed up this process of becoming the perfect size that you were created to be. Why not become healthy in the process and learn a way of eating that will sustain this health and body weight for the rest of your life?

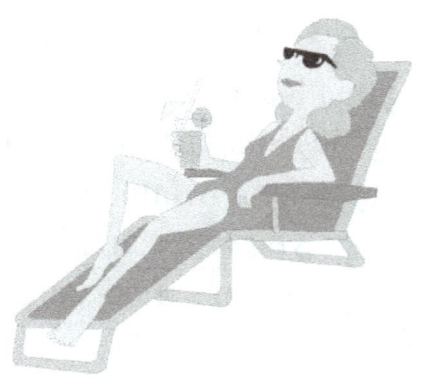

Carbohydrates and Protein

There has been much talk about carbohydrates and protein. There are many low carbohydrate plans with an emphasis on protein. You do lose weight from cutting out carbohydrates, but when you stop your low carbohydrate plan, the body craves it more than ever. We need carbohydrates in the body to keep a balance of sugar. Carbohydrates are a form of fuel for the body. When the body is deprived of them, it burns fat. When the carbohydrates are reinstated, the body craves all that it has been deprived of, trying to get back into the balance it is designed to be in.

Protein is essential for the body to built new cells and renew itself, but too much can overwork the digestive tract and kidneys and clog up the colon.

The best plan is to have a little of both. Again, balance is key. If you don't deprive your body of much needed materials, it won't crave them in excess and get out of balance.

Protein has been given way too much attention. We don't need as much as we've been told we need. All protein drinks are designed for athletes. If you are burning that much energy in working out, you do need protein to rebuild and support your muscle system. If you are not that active, too much protein will overload your system and clog up your digestive tract. This really becomes a very individual decision. As you become a healthy eater, you will know how much protein you need to eat. If you are eating too much, you will become sluggish and constipated. If you're not eating enough or digesting it well, you will feel shaky, light headed, and faint. Your hair and nails will not be healthy looking or strong. Try to experiment with your portions of carbohydrates and protein and find the perfect amount for you.

Calcium

Many of people ask how they will get their calcium if they are not drinking milk or eating a lot of dairy products. We have been somehow convinced that the only place we can get calcium from is dairy. This is not so. There are many other ways to get calcium, and some foods have more calcium than dairy products. Here are some of them:

Oats, sesame seeds, millet, figs, parsley, watercress, green vegetables, eggs, dried fruit, soy beans, boney fish, cereals, and almonds. Almonds, raw and unsalted, contain twice as much calcium as milk (3-1/2 oz. of milk contain 118mg of calcium; almonds contain 234mg of the same quantity).

Water Retention

Some people experience swelling in their bodies, which just exacerbates the feeling of being overweight, or overly conscious of your body size. Too much salt in the body, or an overly toxic system often triggers this. It will be cleared up if you follow the Willing To Change Plan. (You will probably get relief within one week.) Here are some things you can do to get more immediate results:

Parsley is a natural diuretic when made into a tea. Take a bunch of parsley in a gallon of water and simmer it for about 30 minutes. Strain the parsley off and drink the tea throughout the day until you get results.
Celery is also a natural diuretic when made into juice. Juice a bunch of celery with 4 or 5 carrots and have this 2 times a day until you get results.

Here's the Program:

Breakfast

Upon awakening drink one 8-ounce cup of water with a slice of lemon.

Oatmeal with maple syrup-pure, *not* Log Cabin (about 3 T)

You can also use Rice Cereal, Cream of Wheat (all natural…no additives or preservatives), or if you just don't like any of these cereals, the replacement would be a bowl of fruit salad…any fruit except melon-always eat melon alone; it digests best by itself.

Boil 1-1/2 cups of water with a pinch of sea salt. Then add 3/4 cup of instant oatmeal. Let it boil and then cover for about 10 min. (If this is not enough for a man, you can have 2 cups of water with 1 cup of oatmeal.) You can add wheat germ if you like.

If you don't like oatmeal, try any other grain like cream of wheat, or cream of rice.

Snack

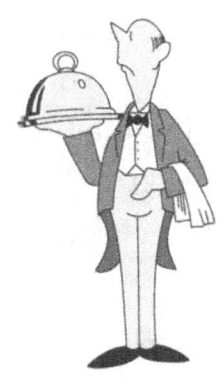

*Fruit salad
    OR
*Carrot Sticks
    OR
*Carrot Juice
    OR

*Rice Cakes with Apple Butter (that has no additives, preservatives, or sugar added…found in health food section of grocery store) *Only if you did not have oatmeal for breakfast!*

Eight ounce glass of water before you eat or one hour after

Make a big bowl of fruit salad with mint leaves (if you like) and keep it for snacks.
You can have 1-1/2 cups of this.

Lunch

Beans and Rice: 1-1/2 cups of brown rice (always use one cup of rice per 2 cups of water, with a pinch of sea salt, bring to a boil, turn down to a simmer and cook for 40-45 minutes), 1 cup of beans (kidney beans, Great Northern Beans, lentils (makes a great soup), lima beans, mung beans (do not need soaking, a very quick, low fat, delicious bean), navy beans, pinto beans, red beans, or soybeans.
Soak beans over night. You can also bring them to a boil right after you put them in water. The longer you soak them, the less gas they will produce. (Sometimes I will soak them for two days.) Frequently change the water. When cooking beans, add one onion and a few cloves of garlic. This also will cut the gas way down. When cooking the beans, occasionally take the foam off the top of the pot of boiling water. This will help you to digest the beans and keep you from experiencing gas.

If you cannot do the beans at all (after trying them, please), then just eat the rice without the beans. (You will be fine without protein for two weeks!) This program is actually more cleansing without the beans. The beans are there to give you protein and sustenance. And because beans are so healthy and whole, they do not take away from the cleansing effect. But some people just can't do beans. If you can get organic chicken, this would be an okay substitute. The cleanse will work best without the chicken. It will still work with the chicken, but will be more effective without. Some people just have to have protein, so this will be an alternate substitute. I'd rather you succeed, and find a way that works for you rather than not do it at all because you don't like beans!

Salad with low fat dressing (one from the health food section in your grocery store)

Eight ounce glass of water before you eat or one hour after

Cook a big pot of beans to have in the refrigerator. Soak overnight, pour out water and add new water, three times the amount of the beans. Cook for 2 or 3 hours with onions and garlic if you like, which cuts down the effects of gas. Have one cup of beans and one cup of rice with tamari or Bronner's Broth. Both of these items are sold at health food stores or the health food section in your grocery store.

Dinner

Stir fry vegetables with a little olive oil, garlic, onion, broccoli, tamari, green pepper, carrots, any herbs such as dill, parsley, basil, oregano, etc, and tomatoes (optional), with brown rice,* 1 1/2 cups.

Salad with low fat dressing

Eight ounce glass of water before you eat or one hour after

*Brown rice is said to calm the nervous system, relieve depression, and strengthen the internal organs. In modern nutrition, it is recommended for those who need extra B vitamins due to stress-related deficiencies. Brown rice is rich in complex carbohydrates, low in fat, and packed with vitamins, minerals, amino acids, and fiber. And it's inexpensive! Brown rice is very balancing to the system. In these first two weeks, this will be our foundational grain.

Evening Snack

Fruit Salad

Any piece of fruit

(Stop eating before 9:00.)

Eight ounce glass of water

Alternative snacks

*Popcorn with garlic powder (not more than 2 cups)

*Rice cakes with apple butter (without preservatives or sugar)…not more than three

*Herb tea with small amount of honey (hot or cold)

*Carrot sticks, cucumber sticks

*Any kind of fresh vegetable juice (the more of this the better; if you do not have a juicer, you can buy bottled

juice in the health food section of your grocery store…make sure it has no added sugar or preservatives)

*Salad with low fat dressing

*Baked sweet potato with a touch of maple syrup

Alternative Lunches

*Corn on the cob (1 cob), salad with low fat dressing

*Steamed broccoli and carrots

*Baked squash, salad with low-fat dressing

*Brown rice with tamari or Bronner's Broth

Alternative Dinners

*Vegetable Stew--one cup (see attached recipe)
Brown rice – 1 ½ cups
Salad with low fat dressing ("Annie's" is a good
one…Kroger sells it in the health food department)

*Lentil Soup

*Any of the vegetable soups
(attached recipes)
Brown rice
Salad with low fat dressing

*Steamed green beans
Brown rice with tamari or
Bronner's Broth
Baked butternut squash

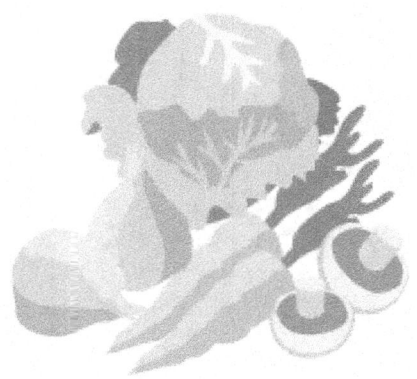

Herbal Teas

Drinking decaffeinated teas can be a great way to give yourself something to do between meals and before you go to sleep. Chamomile is a wonderful relaxant before bed.

Juicing

If you have a juicer, this would be an extremely helpful supplementation to this plan. Juicing is a very powerful way to get high quality nutrition to your cells with the least amount of digestive effort from the body. This will give you more energy and will help heal anything that needs healing in your body. I recommend carrot juice as the number one all around healer and nutritious supplement. You can add parsley and celery to the carrot juice, making it even more nutritious.

Juicing will also fill you up between meals and curb hunger. The more our cells are fed, the less we crave to be filled by food. If you would like to try juicing without investing a lot of money, Walmart or K-mart sells very inexpensive juicers. If you like the effect of juicing, you could then invest in a more quality machine.

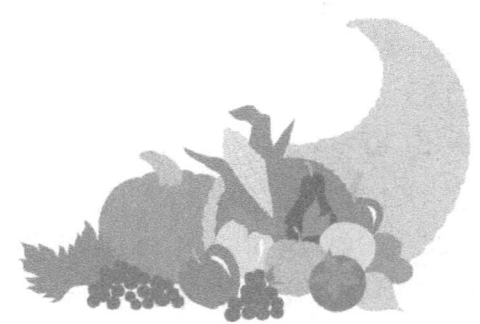

Willing To Change-Level II

After the two weeks of cleansing, you can now begin to add foods that are a little harder to digest. The plan will basically stay the same. What will change is the addition of new foods. These food additions can be substitutions for the original plan meal choices. If your weight begins to level out once you start adding these foods, I would suggest going back to the first level until you start to see some weight loss again. (This doesn't necessarily happen unless you are simply eating too much food and not exercising enough.) Depending on how quickly you would like to lose weight is how long you would want to stay on the first level Willing To Change Cleansing Plan. The simpler you keep your plan, using foods that are quickly and easily digested, the faster you will lose weight. It is not hard to stay on the first Willing To Change level, because you will find that you will not be hungry. The food will satisfy you. You will also be healing your body, your mind will become clearer, you'll have much more energy, and your health will begin to improve dramatically… this can be a motivating factor that will keep you dedicated to your goal of losing weight.

Adding new tastes and diversity will keep you from becoming bored. At this point also, if you slip and eat something that is not on the plan, it will not affect you adversely or keep you from losing weight. The two weeks was a foundational time of preparing and training your body to be in a mode of cleansing and healing. Your body adjusts and cooperates very quickly when given the right kinds of foods. It immediately begins to operate like it was designed to. As long as you go back, as quickly as possible (the next meal, or the next day) to the foundational Willing To Change Plan, whatever you ate will be quickly cleansed and out of your system within twenty-four hours. *It helps to drink more water after eating hard to digest foods.*

It is important to remember to keep as close as possible to the original two-week Willing to Change program while you are in the process of losing weight. You can become more diverse in your food choices, but still maintain a discipline of three balanced meals of suggested portions, with two small snacks a day. *The exercise must continue.* The most success you will achieve will be based on the combination of both changes in your plan and how you exercise. These two aspects of lifestyle changes will bring success.

The Level II Willing to Change Program is very closely aligned with the Beginning Foundational Willing To Change Cleansing Program.

The only difference between the two is the addition of a handful of foods that were not included in the Willing To Change Cleansing Program. These foods are a little heavier and harder to digest. They are healthy and whole, so the body will continue to heal and lose weight. If you find that you are not losing weight as quickly as before, I highly suggest going back to the Level I for a time until you feel comfortable enough to move into Level II again.

Sometimes if you just increase the amount of aerobic exercise you do in one week, this would be enough to keep the weight loss process at an accelerated level without having to go back to the Level I Cleansing Program.

Forgive Yourself

I must interject at this point how important it is to forgive yourself quickly for eating foods you decided you weren't going to eat. Old habits die hard sometimes. Especially in the American culture, with all the temptations, advertisements, fast food places, it can be difficult to eat differently (not to mention peer pressure). Often times people do not want you doing what they are not willing to do. Rather than have themselves feel bad for not eating, people would rather get you to break down and eat something that would make them feel more comfortable. This is where you must pull on your commitment to staying on this plan until you are at your perfect weight (or for at least twenty-eight days, which is how long it takes to implement a new habit). You will become stronger and more stable the longer you stick to your goal. As you experience the benefits of this plan, the more you will have reason to reject the temptations.

The importance of forgiveness in the regard to what you eat cannot be stressed enough. Many times people who do overeat do so because of feelings of unworthiness, dissatisfaction with themselves, and disappointments with themselves for failed goals, dreams, etc. So to feel bad and get mad at yourself for eating the wrong food will only spiral you into negativity that will be counterproductive. It will be very important at this time to quickly forgive, forget, and move on. Accept yourself as human. What will change you and guarantee your success is your willingness to get up and do it again. Get back on the horse, and don't look back!

You will have great success if you can change the way you think about yourself and eating. Beginning this program is an excellent way to start. Make a decision within yourself that you will only think of yourself as a healthy eater continuously on the road to your perfect weight, free from food. Do not leave any room for any other thoughts about yourself in relationship to food and weight. If you can make this one decision, you will absolutely reach your goal of your perfect weight and be free from the bondage of food forever!

Willing To Change-Level II

New Food Substitutions

(Have only *one* piece of bread/muffin per day.)

Breakfast

*1 or 2 hard-boiled eggs (only eat one yoke), preferably free range chicken eggs
1 piece of whole wheat bread, preferably bought at health food store (or health food section in grocery store)
1 glass of carrot juice

OR

*2 or 3 pancakes (made with whole wheat flour--recipe in back of book)
Cooked in very small amount of olive oil with 1 or 2 tlbs maple syrup
(Add blueberries if you'd like.)

OR

*Fruit salad with low fat or nonfat yogurt with small amount of honey or maple syrup (this can also be a good snack or lunch)

Snacks

*Any fruit or vegetable

***Smoothie-** frozen fruit (frozen section of grocery store...black cherries, blueberries, mangos, strawberries, pineapple, peaches), freeze some bananas (peel banana, break in small pieces and put in freezer bag), low fat soymilk, or low fat yogurt, protein powder (optional) sweetened only with 2 T honey or 2 T of maple syrup

*Whole Wheat Muffins-- (recipe in back of book) made with maple syrup, honey or rice syrup (just   **one** for a snack with apple butter)

*Plain Rice Cakes with Apple Butter (all natural with no additives, preservatives, or sugar added)

Lunch

*Salad with *lean chicken strips, or very lean steak strips **(3) (These can be grilled or broiled after marinating in 1 or 2 T olive oil and tamari with some dried basil, dill, and thyme.)

Low fat dressing

* I must interject here that the longer you can keep chicken and beef out of your plan, the faster you will lose weight. These are very hard to digest, and animals are raised these days with a lot of fat in their flesh. Easier digestion with less fat will bring greater results in weight loss (not to mention the many chemicals and hormones that are added to prolong shelf life and keep diseases off of the animals). If you must have meat, this plan will still work…it's just faster without meat.

If you are trying to heal from some type of sickness, I recommend staying away from meat and chicken until you are completely healed. As your body strengthens and you are at your desired weight, it will always be okay to eat meat or chicken. Just keep it in moderation, and you will stay at your perfect weight and health. I put the meat at lunchtime because this will give your body time to digest it the rest of the day. It would not be good to eat at dinner because most people are not very active after dinner, and this could slow the body's production down.

*Chicken noodle soup (recipe in the back of the book) 2 Cups
　　Salad with low fat dressing

Dinner

 *Broiled fish (salmon, tuna, shark, etc.) cooked in tamari, olive oil, herbs, lemon (recipe in the back of the book)
　　Brown rice
　　Steamed broccoli and carrots

*Salad with low fat dressing
　　Stir fried vegetables with whole wheat noodles

*Stir-fried vegetables with lean chicken pieces, or low-fat tofu (after marinating in tamari and a little sesame oil) with sesame seeds on top
　　Brown rice
　　Salad with low fat dressing

*Black bean soup (recipe in back of book)
　　Brown rice
　　Salad

 If you are feeling rather strong and believe you could handle some homemade cookies (made with honey, maple syrup, or rice syrup and wheat flour), you could give yourself a nice treat, as long as you only have a few and believe you could stop at that. Then you must continue back on the Willing To Change Plan.

Willing To Change-Level III...
Once you are at your
perfect weight!

You can now add many different types of healthy foods. There are links to health food recipes in the back of this book. There are also many recipe books that use only healthy ingredients.

*All types of dried fruit make wonderful snacks. (I don't recommend them while you are trying to lose weight, because they are high in concentrated fruit sugar, which brings lots of extra calories.)

*All kinds of nuts and seeds. (I also don't recommend while losing weight because they are high in fat. The lowest in fat would be sesame seeds and sunflower seeds.)

*Trail mix...mix all the nuts and dried fruit together!

*Carob brownies...recipe in back of book

*Spaghetti with vegetarian meat balls...(found in frozen health food section of grocery store)

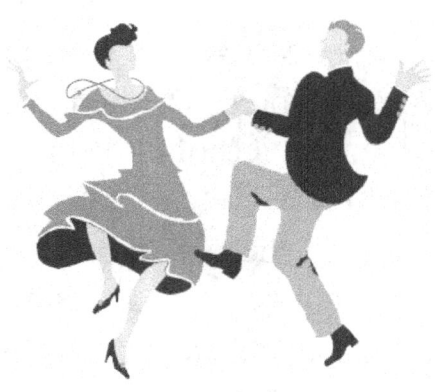

Fasting

Fasting is a great way to accelerate the cleansing process in your body, therefore increasing your body's ability to lose weight. There are all types of fasts. I will give you a few options.

You must know your own limitations at this point in your life as far as what your body can handle when deprived of food. For example, if you have problems with hyperglycemia, or diabetes, I do not recommend a total fast (which is drinking only water for a set period of time). If you have had eating disorders in the past, and are still dealing with this, I would also not recommend a total fast because this could throw you into a binge after being deprived of food. A person dealing with this could do a total fast if they were very secure in knowing they were emotionally free from the compulsion to starve themselves because of severe emotional pain.

Fasting is only recommended for the person who would like to increase the effects of the Willing to Change Plan or who maybe has reached a plateau in his weight loss.

There are three types of fasts that I would like to recommend. They can be done for a period of one to seven days. I will write these fasts in the order that would be best to experiment with them. As you get comfortable with an easier fast, you can move to the next stage of fasting. It is important that you take it in stages, as the body will release toxins at a more rapid pace as you deprive it of food. The body needs to slowly move into adjusting to levels of cleansing in order to have the least amount of side effects. You will then insure your comfort and then succeed in completing your goal.

If you are not used to fasting, I would suggest starting by simply not eating from sunset to sunrise. This is a short and easy fast. Upon arising have a big glass of water and fresh lemon juice. This will acclimate your body towards beginning stages of fasting.

Vegetable and Fruit Fast

The next stage of fasting is just eating vegetables and fruit. Fruit salad can be eaten for breakfast, apple cider (a clean brand from the health food store without additives), water with lemon and plain water in between meals, salad with low fat dressing for lunch, cooked butter nut squash, steamed kale, broccoli, corn, or carrots, and salad for dinner. You can have fruit for snacks if needed. Fresh vegetable juice will add tremendously to the nutritional and cleansing effects of this fast. This is a very healing fast. If you were experiencing any type of sickness, this fast would bring healing to the body because it feeds the cells very quickly without any stress to the body. This fast is a very do-able fast. You will feel very energized and refreshed after this fast whether it is one or two, or seven days.

Juice Fast

Another fast is a juice fast. This is best done with fresh vegetable juice. You can also use apple cider when in season. The best quality would be a brand that did not add chemicals, sugar, or any artificial substances. This fast consists of drinking only juice and water from one to seven days. Also you drink several glasses of plain water and water with fresh lemon juice each day of the fast.

Juicing is an excellent way to heal from many sicknesses. It is a powerful way to put much-needed nutrients into the body without putting any stress on the body for digestion. A lot of times when someone is sick, the body is starving for nutrients, but it's too weak to be able to break them down from the food. This is why people lose their appetite when they are sick, because the body needs all the energy it has to fight the illness, and clean it out. It does not want more to do in digesting food. One can heal oneself of most illnesses with a seven-day juice fast. The more juice you can drink in a day, the better. Some illnesses require a longer period of time in juicing. After one day of juice fasting you will notice an instant change in the way you feel. The cells crave nutrition. When we feed them high quality, live raw food, without having to make them work, they rejuvenate.

Total Fast

The last stage of fasting that I would recommend for the purpose of weight loss and cleansing is called a Total Fast. This is where you drink just water and do not eat any food. This type of fasting is best done when you have a lot of practice with the vegetable and fruit fast, or the juice fast.

You can start with this fast by doing it for just one day. As you get stronger in you ability to fast, you can increase the days. This gives your body a total rest from digestion. This is excellent for your internal organs. There has been much documented about this type of fasting that you can do greater research on. Because this gives the body such a sabbatical from food, it can really do some major deep cleaning within the organs that can have a radical effect of healing on the body. The more you fast, the better you get at it. You also get better at knowing how to move into a fast and how to come off of one with an easy take off and smooth landing. *The more you fast, the freer you get from food.* It's a powerful way to break cycles of addiction and to master the desires of the flesh.

Beginning the fast

You can start fasting by fasting one meal during your day. You can then move into trying two meals. Always moving slowly. Never be upset with yourself if you cannot make it. Just try again another day. If you find that fasting propels you into wanting to binge, then it is not for you at this time (unless you make a practice of it until you master the ability to control yourself after a fast!). Binging will be counterproductive to the benefits of the fast.

The day before a fast it is a good idea to start cutting back your intake of food. Begin increasing your intake of water. Focus on your commitment to begin a fast at the desired set day. Write down when you will end your fast. (Or if it is just one day, commit within yourself to fast one entire day until bedtime). The day you begin your fast, remind yourself of how good you are going to feel when your fast is over. Let yourself know that there is an ultimate goal of losing weight and optimum healing involved. Remember, you will begin to feel clearer and better just after one half day of fasting. There are many books written about the benefits of fasting. It is an excellent thing to do for your body.

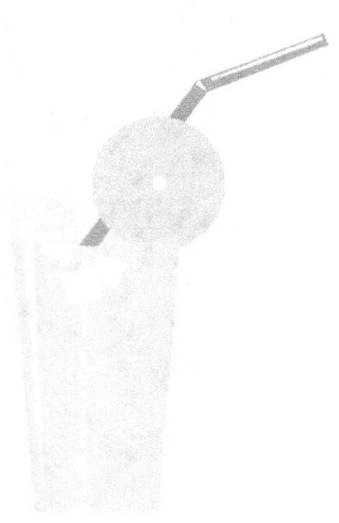

Coming off of a fast

It is important that you come off of a fast slowly so that you do not gorge on what you felt deprived of. Gorging will only bring more stress and imbalances to your body. (This is why a lot of people gain more weight after a plan…they felt deprived so they make up for it when they are off of the plan.) The main truth you need to keep in the forefront of your mind is BALANCE! Fasting is done for the intention of accelerating weight loss and bringing cleansing and health to the body. If it is too hard to do without binging, it is best left alone.

As you come off of a fast, it is best to increase your food intake slowly. This is the way you will get the optimum effects of fasting. This is the way you will also keep your cravings at bay, and keep an upper hand in your ability to control yourself. Remember you are always working on strengthening your will to control your body. You master your body. Do not let it lead you.

The first day after a fast, eat lightly. With each meal you can begin to add more and more of the foods you were not eating. It would be best to just follow the Foundational Willing To Change Plan, Level I. For example, make your first meal smaller than usual, the next meal a little bigger until you are at the normal serving of the Foundational Plan. Wait at least one or two days before adding foods from the Willing To Change Level II Plan.

Plateaus Of Weight Loss

If you find yourself coming to a place where you are staying at the same weight and are not continuing to lose weight, here are some suggestions:

First try a one day a week Vegetable and Fruit fast. Try doing two days the next week. One whole week of just vegetables and fruit will certainly break any plateaus of stubborn weight loss. If this is still not doing it for you, try the Total Fast for one day a week, and then increase it to two days a week (after trying the Vegetable and Fruit fast for one week…and not having results).

Another suggestion is to increase the intensity and frequency of your exercise program. If you are walking for exercise, try jogging or getting a mini trampoline. Aerobic exercise is a proven fat burner. If you are not getting enough, you will not burn fat very quickly.

Cut back on your grain consumption. If you have moved to the Level II Willing to Change Plan, go back to Level I. If you are still at a plateau, eat less fruit and more vegetables. Eat more salads and less cooked food.

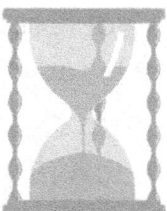

Exercise

There are many types of exercise. I have been experimenting for many years with many areas of exercise. I am going to give you the most effective way that I know works and is the most easily attained. I am going to keep it as simple as possible as I know most people are so confused as to what to do, they have decided not to do any exercise because it's just too complicated.

The most effective type of exercise is the combination of Aerobic and Strength exercise working together. Aerobic exercise would be anything from walking fast, jogging, swimming, stair stepping, aerobic classes, bike riding, skiing, tennis, basketball, soccer, or football, etc. Strengthening is weight training, yoga strength exercises, Karate strength exercises, Palates, or anything that builds the muscles all over the body.

I recommend aerobic exercise 3 to 4 times a week, for at least 20 minutes. If you can do it everyday, that would accelerate your progress immediately. The other 3 days I highly recommend strength exercises.

Aerobic exercise

If you are new to exercise, the best way to start is to begin walking around your block in your neighborhood, town, or city. If you can find a high school track, this is also very good. Start walking every day, or every other day when you get up in the morning, before you start work, or whatever you do for the day. (This way it is out of the way, and you won't procrastinate doing it. Usually it never happens then.) Get into a routine. Then begin to increase your pace little by little until you are at a very fast walk. The whole idea is to get your heart pumping for a good 20 minutes. If you are more experienced, try running (after walking for a bit of warm up). If this is not working for you, get a bike. (This is my personal favorite.) Bike riding in a beautiful park or place where there are bike trails is a healthy, wonderful treat for your mind and spirit. It does amazing things for any kind of stress. There is also swimming at your local YMCA, running on a running machine, stair stepping, classes in aerobics, or, if your legs and back need special care, I highly recommend getting a little trampoline and running in place on it for 20 minutes. This will not put any pressure on your knees or back. A trampoline is easy to store, and you will always have access to it.

Strengthening Exercise

This is a way to strengthen every part of your body. Sometimes if someone is just doing aerobic exercises, one part of their body, like their calves will tone. Strengthening exercise is a way to insure that you will lose weight and tone in the areas you desire. Strengthening and toning the muscles help the body to burn calories more quickly. The more muscle mass you have on your body, the faster you burn calories. (The more you will be able to eat!) Strengthening exercises can be done with weights, or by old fashioned sit-ups, pushups, and leg lifts. (This is really the most simplistic way to get your strengthening exercises done.) Then if you buy some small weights, you can add some arms exercises. I also use Palates, which is a great way to get all of your body toned. (It is based on sit-ups and leg exercises…all designed to strengthen your stomach, leg and back muscles.) This is a very effective form of exercise, and you can do it in 20 minutes. I just follow a video that you can find in most stores, or you can take a class at your local YMCA.

As with the aerobic exercise, I suggest doing your strength exercise first thing in the morning, three times a week. If you are new to exercise, start small and then increase the amount of sets. Begin by doing 10 sit ups (arms behind head, elbows back, knees bent in the beginning or if you have a weakness in your back), 5 pushups, 10 leg lifts on each side (lie on one side, one arm holding up your head, and lift your leg directly above the other leg while keeping your body straight, try and keep your top foot pointed towards the ground, as this will protect your lower back). The next time that it is strength exercise day, increase the amount by doing one set of 10 sit ups, and then another set of 10 sit ups, one set of 5 pushups, and then another set of 5 pushups, and then one set of 10 leg lifts and then another set of leg lifts, switch to the other side. Increase, as you are able each day until you are doing 50 sit-ups, 50 leg lifts on each side, and 10-15 pushups.

If you are lifting weights, I suggest concentrating on legs, butt and calves one day for one half an hour to forty five minutes, and then the next time it is strengthening day, concentrate on your arms, chest, and stomach. The third day of the week of strengthening should be legs, butt and calves again.

If you are doing a Palates video, just find a beginner video and do that for three days of your week. As you get good at it, find an intermediate video. (You can also find these on the internet through e-bay.)

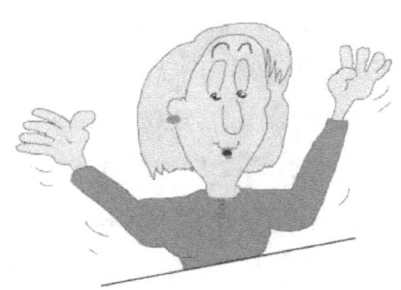

The Importance of Purpose, Creativity, and Inspiration

In my own experience with finding the best way to think about food and eating, I have discovered the important correlation between food, love, purpose, creativity and inspiration. The time in my life that I struggled the most with food, I was depressed, lost and stuck in not knowing why I was here on earth and what I was supposed to do. On top of all that, I was very insecure and full of self-hatred. The only comfort I had was food. (I was involved with other addictions, but I consider food to be just as addicting but harder to be free of because of our need for it to sustain life).

A lot of very creative people have struggles with drugs, alcohol, and food. This is because these substances can often be both stimulating and numbing to these creative forces inside. When we are unsure about what we are to do with our creative urges and desires, we either want to numb them or stimulate them in order to get some relief or release.

God has created us to create. We were created in His image and He is the One and Only Great Creator. (Genesis 1:27…So God created man in His own image, in the image and likeness of God He created him; male and female He created them.) He created us to desire creativity and wants us to satisfy these creative urges. He derives pleasure in our success in creating and completing the purpose that he called us to. He says in His word that He delights in our prosperity (Psalm 35:27…Let the Lord be magnified, Who takes pleasure in the prosperity of His servant.). Prosperity is wholeness and the fulfillment of our desires. When you are in the perfect plan of God (found in your heart through desires that you are naturally drawn to and usually good at), prosperity will come as a result of your walking through and carrying out ideas and creative dreams that He has placed in your heart. God also says that He will give us the desires of our heart (Psalm 38:4…Delight yourself also in the Lord, and He will give you the desire and secret petitions of your heart). God is the one who puts these desires in our hearts. He knows what they are. We simply need to listen to our hearts and discover our God-given purpose. A lot of times people are unsure what these desires are. The best way to find out is to step out on what you think they are. This will often lead you to what you need to do, or you will find out what it is definitely not!

We all have a purpose to fulfill, and this comes through a desire to satisfy creative urges that have to do with our purpose. Food can be a counterfeit satisfaction to dull or quiet urges of creativity. Food has the ability to bring satisfaction on a very short-term basis to these hungers that we have need of expressing. We are ultimately only satisfying taste buds and bodily hungers for food and food addictions. These hungers are often confused with hunger for the fulfillment of God's plan for your life, especially if you have never been taught about this. Our society is so saturated in food satisfaction, it is easy to be continually distracted and deceived into thinking that all the hunger that you have within you is for food.

The biggest hunger we have is first of all to know our Creator and to love Him. Jesus had said to love God with all your heart and love your brothers and sisters. God is Love. He created us in His image of Love. He sent Jesus to satisfy His intense love for us. (Ephesians 2:4…But God--so rich is He in His mercy! Because of and in order to satisfy the great and wonderful and intense love with which He loved us.) Jesus had to come in order for us to be reconciled back to God the Father.

God is Holy. He cannot look upon sin. When Adam first rebelled by not obeying God's instructions in the garden, he separated us all from God by choosing his own way rather than God's way. God never takes back His word. Once God says something, it is, and it will be fulfilled. He told Adam that he would die (spiritually) if he ate from the tree of knowledge. This meant that he would be separated from God. Then through Moses, God set up the law through the Ten Commandments and designed a way that man could cleanse himself from his sin (which defines itself as disobedience through worshipping his own self or other gods) through the sacrificing of animals. This way man could then come closer to God to fellowship with God as Moses often did. But God wanted another way for man to come back to Him without the need for sacrifice. (For You delight not in sacrifice, or else would I give it: You find no pleasure in burnt offering. Psalm 51:16. ...Has the Lord as great a delight in burnt offerings and sacrifices as in obeying the voice of the Lord? Behold, to obey is better than sacrifice, and to hearken than the fat of rams. 1 Samuel 16.) He had to find a way to bring man back to Himself because He loves us and wants us so much to be with Him. He created a way that would once and for all end the need to sacrifice animals or the need to follow after ridged laws one would have to perform to be clean. (There were many acts that appointed priests would have to go through in order to spend time with God. They would always tie a rope to the priest's leg when they went into the Holy of Holies…a temple that was built for God…because if he was not clean enough through sacrifice or whatever else he had to do, he would die in the presence of God.)

God cannot look on sin. He is Holy. His power is so intense, that without a covering or washing of our sin, we cannot live and be in His presence. That was why

Moses was the only one that was willing and able to speak with God. He set himself apart and followed God completely through all that he needed to do to be in God's presence. God's followers, the Israelites, did not want to go close to the mountain when God spoke to Moses because it was too overwhelmingly painful to their souls. We are ever conscious of our unholiness when we are in the presence of God.

So God sent Jesus, His only Son, to come to earth and lay down His Godhood, become a man so that He could suffer the consequences of all man's sin. (John 3:16 *For God so greatly loved and dearly prized the world that He gave up His only begotten Son, so that whoever believes in Him shall not perish (come to destruction, be lost) but have eternal (everlasting life).* Therefore all of God's word had been fulfilled. All He asks us to do is believe that Jesus died for us, take Him as our sacrifice through repenting of all our sins, and receive Him as Lord of our life. (This means we will look to Him always for guidance and direction.)

He desires us to Love Him. He wants our Love, just like we want His love. We are just like Him in love. The love and the desire to create have been put in you to compel you to fulfill the plan God has for you. He gave us all gifts. Every one of us has a gift or gifts from God that need to be developed and expressed. They are there for a purpose and are a part of the great purpose that He created us for. He wants us to be a part of His creating. To love God, love each other and create like God creates is His gift to us. When we desire to give what we create and seek from God, what it is that would please Him for us to create, this is our gift and love back to God.

If you don't have a clue what your particular gift and ultimate purpose is, or have a lot of creative drive and no outlet, the tendency is to try and satisfy this desire with food or substance. The devil has perverted the whole plan just like he did in the garden when he tempted Adam and Eve to eat from the tree that God had told them not to eat from.

Deciding to lose weight can sometimes not be enough of a motivating force to overcome deep-seated habits of filling unidentified needs, especially when one has learned how to live around and with habits of addiction. When one has figured out a way to cover up his overweight body in an acceptable way for himself, he can maintain a copasetic life. This secret love affair with food can cover up dreams, ambitions, and a desire for love that will never be uncovered unless the addiction is identified, exposed, and brought to an end.

Food As a Creative Source

Food is very creative, sensual, comforting, warming, satisfying, and very addictive. Women have been known to crave chocolate, when what they really need is love and attention. There actually are chemicals in chocolate that trigger the brain to sensuality and creativity, plus stimulants that trigger needs for closeness and comfort.

What I'm trying to get you to see is that one must identify in themselves a desire to recognize their own dreams, desires, and creativity. This will lead one on the road to his or her own purpose. This is extremely important in order to gain the ambition and driving force needed to break addictions to food (or any other substance for that matter). You will never have to battle with this again if you discover what it is you have a passion for and go for it with all that you have. Food will never have power over you again.

The way to simply begin this journey is to ask God, "In the name of Jesus, what is it that you created me for? Lead me now in uncovering the desires and dreams that you have placed in my heart." (Jeremiah…I know the plans I have for you, plans to prosper you...)

We need to ask ourselves some tough questions. Do I like myself? Do I love myself? Do I feel lovable or loved? Do I think God loves me? Can I open up to His love? Am I willing to trade food for God?

Most people don't have any idea that they are numbing themselves with food. They have done it for so many years that they have let go of any hidden desires or dreams. They have believed lies about themselves. Lies they heard from other people and lies they have heard from society and believed. God's word holds the only truth. And in His word He tells us over and over how much He loves us and how valuable we are to Him. This is the underlying power that we must base our freedom upon. It is no man, thing, person, place or thought other than... "God loves us and wants us to believe this!" When we open up to His love we can open the door to a new way of looking at ourselves, God and this world we live in. We are no longer tied to controlling thoughts of bondage. We are no longer boxed into stereotypes, styles, or what is expected of us. We move into the realm of why we were created, and how important we are to God's whole design. We open up to our part of this amazing plan and beauty of God. Food becomes necessary and fun rather than bondage or something that steals all our time and thought life.

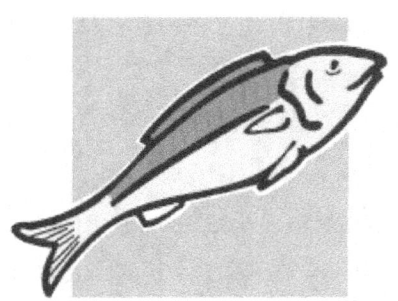

Dieting Versus The Willing To Change Way of Eating

The best kept secret about The Willing To Change way of eating is that you can eat a lot and not gain weight. Foods that are clogging and are hard to digest are what put weight on the body. Examples are white flour, fried foods, lots of fatty meats, processed meats and cheeses, white sugar, and lard.

The problem with dieting is that it creates a dichotomy within us that begins to develop patterns of habits. The habit is I'm either on a diet, or I'm not. If I'm on a diet, I am restricted. I'm in a frame of mind that says I'm on a diet. Now this can mean a lot of different things to different people. Most people's flesh rebels within, and we begin to become irritable and angry and feel deprived. The stronger part of you usually will calm this down by telling yourself, "This will soon be over, and when it is, you can have all that you desire!" So you hold on in anticipation for the desired results of weight loss. When the diet is over, the flesh has a party, indulging itself in all the forbidden fruit (so to speak). Now you have yourself in a black and white situation. Now that you've binged for awhile, you probably need to go on a diet. And the guilt and shame can be overwhelming to some people, compounding the desire to bury oneself in food in order to numb these feelings.

I used to live like this. This can become so debilitating because there is not peace in it. It takes so much time away from your thought life that could be spent on more productive endeavors. The Willing To Change way of eating has been developed through much research, experimentation, experience, and much prayer. God has led me to the revelation, understanding and wisdom of eating healthy, balanced meals of whole foods, with whole food snacks, and it has brought peace in my life with food. I can eat what I want, when I want, and sometimes weeks at a time I will eat lots of junk food (when on vacation usually), and I never gain weight because I always come back to my basic plan of whole foods. I have to add that I am desiring to not eat too much food that has no benefit to my body, because I enjoy how good I feel when I don't. (This was definitely not the norm for me in the past…I was very obsessed with food and was either eating or thinking about eating all the time). This desire decreases more and more as I come into greater revelation and understanding of how much the Father God, through Jesus Christ, loves me.

When I do not eat the best food for a period of time, I become irritable, tired, and sluggish. After eating better for one to three days (depending on how pure I eat), I feel like myself again. I feel energized, light, and ready to do whatever it is I need to do.

When you learn to eat this way, you no longer have to go on diets. You spend less time thinking about food, your weight, and how you look. You know you are doing the best possible thing you can for your body through food. And if you want more out of your food, you can simply add higher quality foods like organic vegetables and fruit, supplements (which I will go into later), and green drinks. You can exercise more; get outdoors more, and you will notice more energy and a better sense of well being. You can enjoy parties with lots of yummy food and celebrate with family and friends without any guilt because you have found a way of eating that you know is sustaining you in good health. I believe in being free in life, especially in the area of food. A lot of so called healthy eating people are so bound up by their healthy eating that I think it is actually taking away from their life because they put too much thought time into it. They are still in obsession; it's now about eating only healthy food, but they are still in fear about not being okay if they do not eat the right things. They have not identified the root problem which is not feeling loved by their heavenly Father. This is only attained by a personal relationship with Jesus Christ. Even Jesus said, "Isn't life much more than food and drink?" (Matthew 6:25) I believe that if you can change your whole attitude and outlook on food, you can be completely delivered from all the adverse effects that food can have on the body. When you do not have a healthy relationship with food, you will not get the ultimate benefits from eating high quality food because your thinking is all messed up about it. All things change from the inside out. In order to receive health benefits from food, you must eat it with the attitude of a decision to be healthier, not out of fear that you are "bad" if you don't. Then you will resent eating right because you have to in order to not be "bad". If you eat healthily while resenting it, your thought will prevent it from having an awesome benefit to your body. The idea here is to think right about food…from the inside out. Then what's on the inside will manifest itself on the outside. If you see eating healthy as being deprived, you will never move past binging to fulfill the loss your flesh and mind experienced. You need to think, "I have decided to change my mind about my relationship to food (hence the name Willing To Change), I am going to learn how to eat what will benefit my life and everyone around me. I am going to enjoy eating healthy, and I'm going to do what it takes to learn how to shop and prepare food that is good for me."

For example, when you get yourself on the Willing To Change way of eating, you can eat a candy bar, enjoying it, knowing it will be cleaned out from the body easily and efficiently, and it will! If you eat a candy bar with all kinds of guilt and condemnation, first of all, it won't be enjoyable, and then it will have a negative effect on the body because of the stress associated with your thought towards yourself for eating it.

"The Willing To Change Program is most effective if it is looked at as a change in the way you eat and look at food. This combined with exercise is a definite guarantee of permanent weight loss, health, and high quality of life."

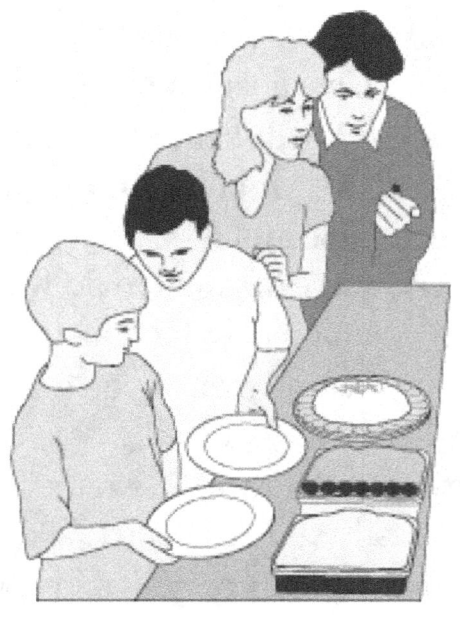

Going To Parties

When you are at a party, you could possibly eat just the fruits and vegetables. (You have really gained power over the flesh!) This of course would be the optimum suggestion especially if you trying to lose weight in an accelerated amount of time or are in your first two weeks of cleansing on the Willing To Change Program. It would be okay to have a *little* of the dip on the veggies and fruit. The key is being a little! I've seen friends of mine at restaurants or parties, who tell me they can't seem to lose weight and all they eat are fruits and vegetables (I'm already suspicious), pour lots of salad dressing and dip like there is no tomorrow. Some of these salad dressings have more than 20 grams of fat per tablespoon!

If you are not in a place of needing to lose weight rapidly, or are in the first two weeks of The Willing To Change Program, go ahead and have a treat at the party…as long as you commit to going back to the Willing To Change Program the following day. The trick is knowing what you can handle. For some people, eating something their new eating program in the beginning state is enough to send them into a three day binge! You have to know yourself well in this area. Sometimes this takes a few times of experiencing yourself, believing you can handle it and then finding out you're not strong enough yet. A lot of times food at parties is just not that good anyway. And in the long run, it is just not worth the effect it has on you the next day as far as your energy level and what you have accomplished so far on your new way of eating. I've come to the conclusion within myself that only the home baked treats are ever worth it to me. I suggest you pick one thing that you believe is worth it to you. Once you make a decision about this, you'll always have it to fall back on when you find yourself in party situations. This will cut down on the quantity of food you eat and keep you on top of your flesh. Every opportunity you give to the flesh to do what it wants opens more opportunity for it to be less disciplined. It is amazing what one little decision made within ourselves will do to help us stay on course. Also when we eat a lot of different fatty foods that we are not used to at one time, it really bogs the body down because it has to break down a lot of foreign substances all at once.

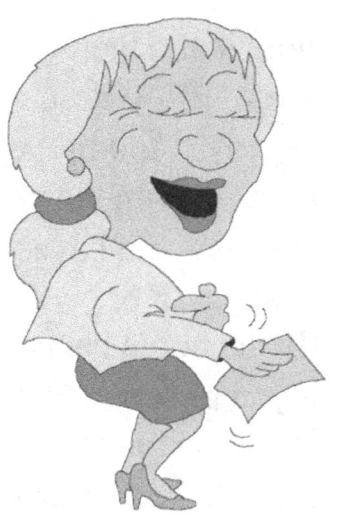

Shopping List For First Two Weeks Of Cleansing

Health Food Store

(Some of these items can be found in the health food section of your grocery store.)

Brown rice- sometimes less expensive in the bulk section of your nearest health food store.

Tamari- pure soy sauce made from soybeans and sea salt. Soy sauce sold in the grocery store is full of chemicals and is watered down. Tamari is very rich and tasty. It can be used for an array of recipes.

Bragg's liquid aminos- this can be used as a replacement to Tamari. It has minerals in it and is best used after food has been cooked, as heat will destroy the good benefits of the minerals and vitamins in this. It is very good for your health.

Rice cakes-try and buy the ones without added sugar or chemicals. Plain is best.

Apple Butter-without sugar or chemicals.

Sesame seeds- usually in the oriental section of grocery stores or health food stores. These are yummy on salads or in stir fry. (Recipes in back of book)

Grocery Store Shopping

Vegetables -Best would be to find a local farm in spring, summer or fall! In your grocery store, pick out the vegetables that look the most vibrant and color filled. Organic is always best but not necessary. If you can afford them, get them. If not, it's perfectly fine to not have organic. Remember, your body is designed to clean out!

Garlic, onions, carrots, kale, corn, mushrooms, lettuce, cucumbers, tomatoes, sprouts, avocados (after losing the weight you desire…these are high in fat), artichokes, asparagus. cauliflower, collards, endive, Jerusalem artichokes, leeks, okra, parsnips, parsley, rutabaga, rhubarb, turnips, watercress, frozen peas, lima beans, celery, potatoes (sweet and regular potatoes), winter squash (acorn, butternut, hubbard, pumpkin), summer squash (yellow, spaghetti, zucchini), artichokes, brussel sprouts, string beans, beets…beet greens, a variety of fresh greens for salad, sprouts, corn, etc. Anything that is a vegetable!

Fruits- Bananas, oranges, kiwi, grapefruit, grapes, pineapples, mangoes, strawberries, blueberries, raspberries, cranberries, cherries, dates, figs, melon, cantaloupe, honeydew, watermelon (melons are best eaten alone), papayas, plantain, plums, pomegranate, prunes, tangerines, pears, peaches, etc. Any kind of fruit!

Herbal teas -any kind as long as it's pure without caffeine or added chemicals. Green tea is okay as it has less caffeine than black tea.

Honey- raw and unfiltered is best

Herbs and Spices- Basil, bay leaf, cardamom, cayenne, cinnamon, chili powder, coriander, cumin, curry, dill, garlic, ginger root, mustard seed, myrrh, nut-meg, oregano, paprika, parsley, rosemary, sage, tarragon, tumeric, thyme (to name a few)

Olive oil- extra virgin best.

Beans -any kind…black beans, red beans, lentils, split green peas, navy beans, pintos, white beans, etc.

Frozen fruits -any kind as long as it says "just fruit" in the ingredients.

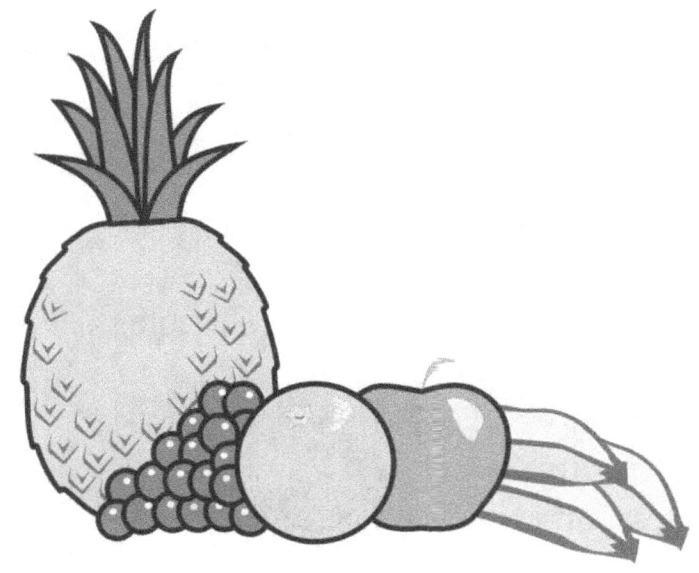

Shopping For Level II-
(After Two Weeks of Cleansing)

Grocery Store-Level II

Eggs-Are best for you if they have been produced by grain fed chickens (without growth hormones and antibiotics…which commercial eggs have in them)

Bread-Buy your bread for now, as you are in the weight loss process, in the health food section of your grocery store, or in the health food store. If you are energetic, you can make your own! Whole grain or whole wheat is best.

Whole Wheat Flour-without any additives or chemicals (This is for making muffins, pancakes, or healthy cookies.)

Chicken- best if grain fed, but grocery store chicken is okay.

Fish-any kind

Beans

Brown Rice

Vegetables-as mentioned Level I Shopping list

Fruit-as mentioned Level I Shopping list

Low-fat yogurt-without sugar or additives

Low fat soymilk-only with natural sweetener added or plain

Whole Wheat, Rice, or any kind of whole grain pasta

Low fat Salad Dressing- usually in the health food department of the Grocery store

Rice Cakes-Plain without any additives, preservatives, or sugar

Health Food Store-Level II

Tamari

Brown Rice in Bulk-Sometimes can be inexpensive this way

Whole Wheat Pasta in Bulk-Also can inexpensive

Whole Wheat or Corn Tortillas

Spaghetti Sauce without added sugar-Can also find this in the health food section of grocery store.

Honey - raw & unfiltered.

Brown Rice Syrup (health food section of grocery store…more expensive than honey, but easier on the body as far as sugar assimilation goes)

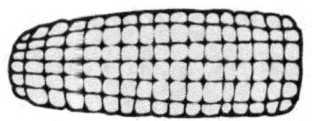

Health Food Store-Level III

After you have reached your goal in losing the weight you desire, you can chose from many types of whole foods creating menus that are delicious, satisfying, nutritious, and low fat. It is important that you stay as close as you possibly can to whole foods and health foods that contain as few ingredients as possible. Remember, the more simple it is for the body to digest, the faster it will be processed through the body with ease, and you will gain the most benefits from it without any weight gain. Every time you eat, you have a choice to make. If you choose wisely more often, overall you will remain healthy and at your perfect size. You will also feel the best you've ever felt and be free from having to worry about your body and food anymore.

Cheese

Cheese can be added in moderation. It is important to use cheese that has not been highly processed. American cheese, cream cheese, or deli cheeses are examples of very processed food. These cheeses are okay every once in a while but try not to make a habit of eating them. They can be clogging to the intestines and colon. The best cheese for the body is made from goat cheese. Goat cheese is easy to digest. Kefir is another cheese that is actually good for you because like yogurt, it is fermented and holds many valuable nutrients that bring healthy enzymes into your digestive tract.

The more health you can bring to the digestive tract, colon and intestines, the better off you are going to be. All food comes through and is broken down through these systems, so if you eat things that are clogging, it will slow your digestion down, and ultimately slow every other system in your body. This is why salad, raw vegetables, fruits, grains, steamed or vegetables made in soup, stews, or stir fries are best for the digestion. These foods are full of nutrients, fiber, minerals, and rich water content, bringing life and health to the digestive tract. They then go through the intestines and colon bringing more nutrients, while the fiber cleanses what needs to be cleaned out.

Meat

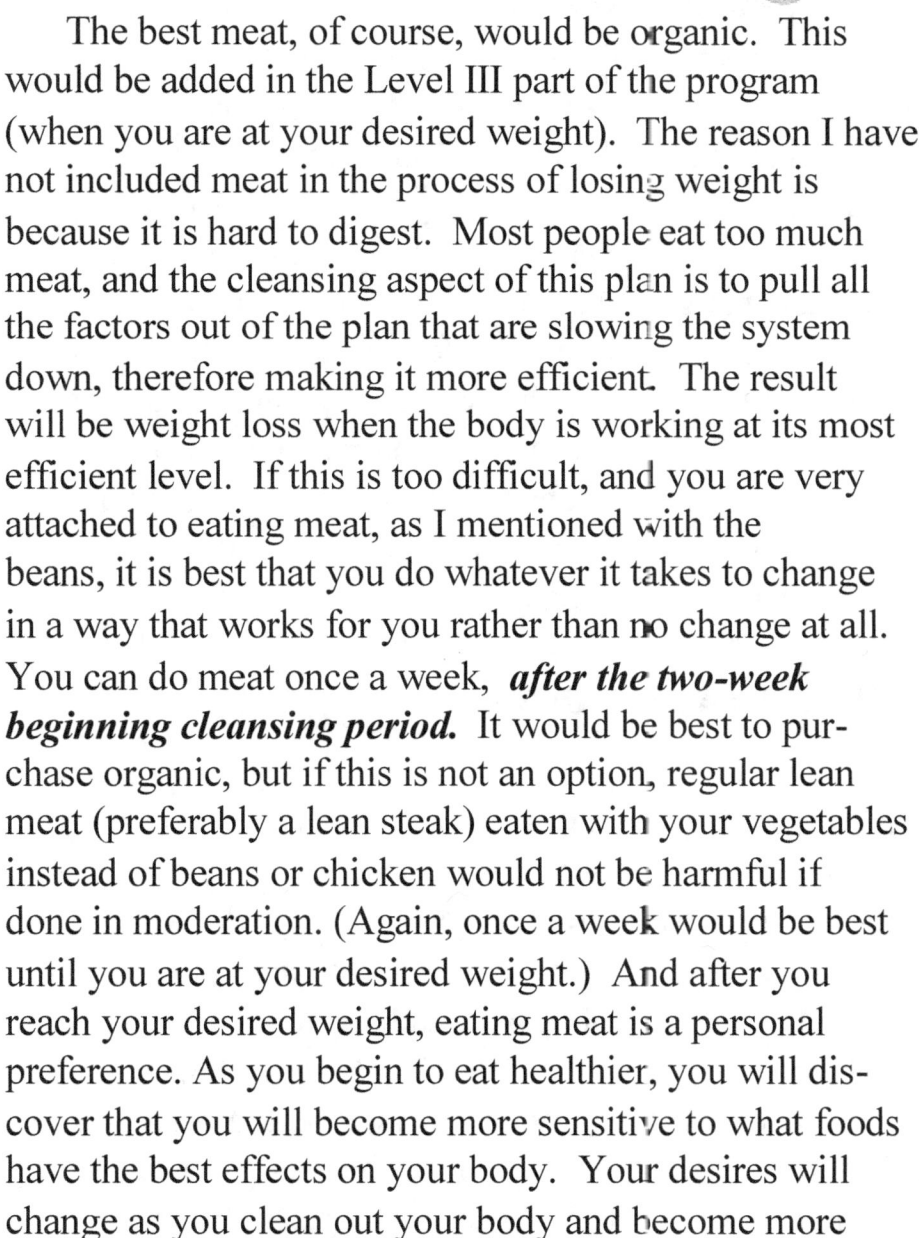

The best meat, of course, would be organic. This would be added in the Level III part of the program (when you are at your desired weight). The reason I have not included meat in the process of losing weight is because it is hard to digest. Most people eat too much meat, and the cleansing aspect of this plan is to pull all the factors out of the plan that are slowing the system down, therefore making it more efficient. The result will be weight loss when the body is working at its most efficient level. If this is too difficult, and you are very attached to eating meat, as I mentioned with the beans, it is best that you do whatever it takes to change in a way that works for you rather than no change at all. You can do meat once a week, *after the two-week beginning cleansing period.* It would be best to purchase organic, but if this is not an option, regular lean meat (preferably a lean steak) eaten with your vegetables instead of beans or chicken would not be harmful if done in moderation. (Again, once a week would be best until you are at your desired weight.) And after you reach your desired weight, eating meat is a personal preference. As you begin to eat healthier, you will discover that you will become more sensitive to what foods have the best effects on your body. Your desires will change as you clean out your body and become more aware of your own eating habits. You will notice the difference, for instance, between cravings that are simply just pleasurable and cravings that are actual needs of the body. Sometimes, I believe, we need a very concentrated form of protein (like meat), and sometimes we need to stay away from it. These needs of the body become more apparent to you as you eat healthier because your body is not clouded and clogged up with all kinds of toxins. It is not so overloaded that it can't "see straight" (so to speak)! So my suggestion is that you do whatever it takes to eat the most balanced plan that you can possibly eat without stressing over what is "bad" and what is "good" for you. *My aim is to help people be free, not put them in more bondage over food.* So find what works for you, and stick to it as your foundational eating plan. Everyone's body works slightly differently, and reacts differently to protein, carbohydrates, and sugars. Some people do better with a little more protein, some do better with less protein, or hardly any, some people do best with less carbohydrates, and some need more (usually if they are more active). So find your balance. Know what works for you. This, you will find, will bring the greatest success in bringing your body to a perfect state of health.

Boxed Dinner Food

Fantastic Foods (found in your health food store, or in the health food section at your grocery store) has great, delicious meals that anyone can create very quickly, inexpensively and easily. They have a chili which you need to only add canned beans (without added chemicals) and canned tomatoes (fresh if you'd like). *Fantastic Foods* also has taco mix, which only needs water added, and Sloppy Joes mix, which only needs canned tomato paste. (It is best to use whole corn tortillas, which can only be found at the health food store or in the health food section of your grocery store.)   All these foods combined with a salad make great quick meals when there is no time to cook.

Boca makes a great soy burger that you can find in the frozen food section of your grocery or your health food store. This put together with some whole grain bread, lettuce, tomato, and healthy ketchup (also sold in the health food section of the grocery or health food store) is delicious.

Salsa- You can get this in the grocery store. Most salsas do not add chemicals. Look for ones without added sugar. You can eat these with tortilla chips that don't have added chemicals. (Best if has just sea salt.)

Oils- Olive oil is always best. Grape seed, avocado, almond are all excellent, but a bit pricey. Sunflower is good for baking and frying tortillas. Canola and safflower are okay. Flax seed oil, fish oil, and omega 3 oil are all wonderful to take as supplements (do not heat these oils as heating will destroy the benefits of the nutrients in them). These oils are especially excellent for women as they are very healing to the hormonal system.

Nuts and Dried Fruits

These are a wonderful snack choice. Bring this into your plan only when you have come to your desired weight. They are healthy, but the dried fruit has lots of concentrated fruit sugar, which adds a lot of extra calories…(good for hikes and lots of exercise), and the nuts have a lot of fat.

Supplements

Good supplements are always an added plus to any plan you are on. For the first two weeks of this program, it is recommended not to take supplements, as this is a cleansing time. Supplements are to build and nourish the body. The first two weeks is dedicated to cleansing and healing the body of excessive toxins. You don't want to add anything to this simple plan for the first two weeks in order to cleanse the system.

Supplements are not necessary if you are eating a healthy plan of vegetables, grains, and fruit. If you are ill, or very tired, it is a good thing to take good quality supplements to add to the plan what may be lacking in vitamins and minerals. Many people claim that because our soil has been depleted by excessive farming and use of chemicals and pesticides that our food lacks the quality of vitamins and minerals that it used to have. This is a very individual choice. If you feel tired all the time after eating The Willing To Change Plan, first try adding juicing to your plan. This is the highest and best way to get live enzymes, vitamins and minerals in your body. If you still lack energy, I would then try green foods like Spirilina, Wheat grass, or Barley Green. These greens would be highly recommended if you need healing in any area of your body. Taking these greens (or juicing, or combining them together) is a sure way to build complete health in your body when you are eating The Willing To Change suggested program. What we're after is the most vibrant type of whole food that has not been processed and is most easily digested by the body. You will get the most out of your money in trying this type of supplementation first. If you still need more vitamins and minerals, the next best for your body, that is assimilated by the body without waste, are vitamins and minerals in either liquid form, or chewable, that have no added chemicals or fillers and are derived from whole foods. Most of the vitamins that you buy at the supermarket are very processed and are synthetic (made chemically, rather than taken from whole foods). I once heard that a man, who worked cleaning those portable bathrooms, saw thousands of vitamins in all of the waste! Synthetic vitamins don't break down in the body so you do not get any benefit out of them at all. You just waste your money. If you want to add supplementation to your plan, in summary:

1. Juicing

2. Green Foods…Barley Green, Spirulina, or Wheat Grass

3. Liquid Vitamins…bought at health food store, or vitamin store without added sugar or chemicals.

4. Chewable Vitamins…Make sure they are sweetened only with fruit juice (fructose), or any type of natural sweetener. I suggest Nature's Plus…Source of Life-Adult's Chewable.

5. High quality Vitamins that are made for easy digestion (usually more expensive)…these are best found by asking in a vitamin store or health food store.

6. Spirulina balls or bars are an excellent snack food. Bettylousinc.com has a very good tasting product. These have a lot of added protein, vitamins and herbs that bring support to your immune system and energy level. I would not have more than one a day after the two week cleanse, because they have almond butter which has a high fat content. If you level out in weight loss, I would increase in exercise or cut these out for a while. Start them in Level II as an added supplement.

Recipes for all Levels

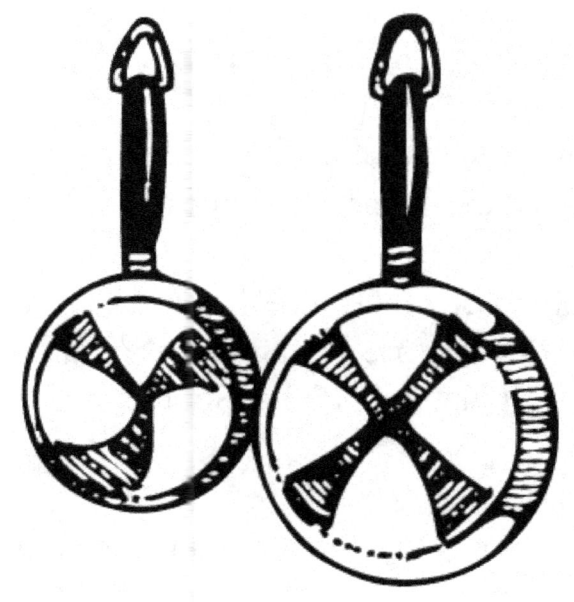

Vegetable Stew (Level I)

2 med onions, sliced
3 cloves crushed garlic
2 medium potatoes, small chunks
3 carrots, sliced
2 stalks celery, sliced
1 eggplant, diced
2 medium small zucchini, in chunks
1 stalk fresh broccoli, sliced

3 fresh tomatoes, diced
1 lb. sliced mushrooms
3 tbs. tomato paste
3 tbs. molasses
1 tsp. dill weed
Tamari to taste
Olive oil for sauté

In a stew pot, begin sautéing onions, garlic, potatoes, and eggplant in olive oil. Add a little tamari and black pepper when potatoes begin to get tender. Add celery, broccoli, and carrots, steam until all vegetables begin to be tender, and then add zucchini, tomatoes paste, tomatoes, mushrooms, molasses, dill and tamari to taste. Simmer over low heat, (20 minutes).

Chicken Soup (Level II)

2 big chicken breasts (skinned before putting in soup)
2 onions
1 half stalk of celery
4 or 5 carrots, chopped
5 cloves of garlic, minced
4 potatoes, cubed
4 Tbsp olive oil
2 bay leaves
1 1/2 Tbsp basil
1 Tbsp dill
1 Tbsp thyme
1 package of whole-wheat egg noodles (should find them in noodle section)
1 or 2 boxes of vegetable broth (if desired from health food section of grocery store)
5 Tbsp of Tamari
Black pepper to taste

Stir fry the chicken in olive oil until browned on every side. Add chopped onions and minced garlic. Keep stir-frying the chicken, garlic and onions until onions are clear. Add chopped celery (as small as you like it), diced carrots, cubed potatoes, and all of the herbs. Stir-fry all vegetables with chicken until all have been slight-ly cooked (continue to stir so that all vegetables get touched by heat and oil). Add broth and water until all the ingredients are covered with 3 inches of water over them. Add Tamari. Cook until potatoes, carrots, and celery are done. Add noodles and cook for another 5-10 minutes. Add more Tamari and pepper to taste. (Canned creamed corn tastes excellent in this soup although I don't recommend it until you are at your desired weight because it does have added sugar).

Stir Fried Vegetables with Rice or Whole-Wheat Noodles

(Level I-Rice, Level II Whole-Wheat Noodles)

This can be made with either chicken, low-fat tofu (or regular Tofu when you are at your perfect weight), Tempeh (found in health food store refrigerator section), or just made with vegetables.

2 carrots
1 onion (or leek, or green onion)
1 stalk of celery
1 package of low-fat tofu (or chicken tenders)
4 cloves of garlic
1 half bunch of broccoli
1 handful of snow peas
1 handful of mung bean sprouts (if desired)
1 half of a green pepper, chopped
1 Tbsp of olive oil
2 Tbsp of Tamari
Pepper to taste

Heat frying pan with olive oil for about 2 minutes to get hot. Start by stir frying the onion and garlic in the olive oil. When onions are clear, add carrots, celery, and green pepper. Stir fry a few more minutes. Then add cubed Tofu. (If making with chicken, before veggies, stir fry cut up chicken, in two inch pieces, until browned all over, cooking in some olive oil with a little garlic and put aside until the end.) Add broccoli, snow peas, mung bean sprouts and Tamari. Use pepper to taste if desired. Serve over rice or whole-wheat noodles.

Carob Brownies (Level III)

1 cup whole wheat or rye flour
2/3 cups chopped walnuts or pecans (optional)
1/2 cup carob (sifted)
1 ½ tsp baking powder
½ tsp sea salt

Blend in a blender:
1 cup rice syrup or honey
2/3 lb melted butter
1 egg
2 Tbsp molasses
1 Tbsp vanilla

Combine all of the above, mixing together thoroughly…Butter an 8x10 inch baking dish and fill with the brownie batter. Bake at 350 for 12 minutes; then remove brownies from the oven and place right into the refrigerator until cool…Slice and serve.

Variation: for a more chocolate-like flavor, try the following:
Mix in a bowl:
1 cup whole wheat or rye flour
2/3 cup chopped walnuts or pecans
1/3 cup cafix (or other coffee substitute)
1 cup carob (sifted)
1 ½ tsp baking powder

2/3 cup honey
2/3 lb melted butter
½ cup molasses
1 egg

Combine and bake the above just like the carob brownies…

Willing to Change

Sue's Sweet Potato Soup (Level I)

4 sweet potatoes
1 bunch of celery
6 cloves of garlic
2 onions
2 zucchinis
1/4 bunch of broccoli
1 cup of barley
½ cup of Tamari
2 tsp of basil
2 tsp of dill
2 tsp of thyme
Black pepper to taste

Cook sweet potatoes by either baking (350 for 45 minutes) or first peeling and steaming them. While sweet potatoes are cooking, put in a soup pot…olive oil, finely chopped celery, chopped onions, minced garlic, chopped zucchinis, and cut broccoli (bite size pieces). Stir fry vegetables until onions are clear. When sweet potatoes are soft, peel them (if you baked them) and put into blender or food processor with enough water to puree them. Puree them until they are creamy. Then add them to the vegetables with more water to have a soup consistency. Add herbs. Add Tamari and pepper to taste. Add the barley and simmer about 30 minutes (until barley is cooked). This soup is delicious with a nice big salad.

*Can add Louisiana Hot Sauce or cayenne pepper if desired.

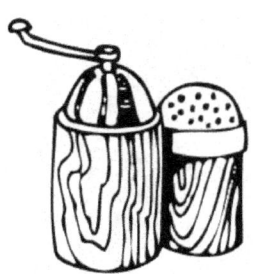

Basic Soup Stocks

The easiest way to always have a supply of soup stock on hand is to save the water when you steam vegetables or boil chicken. This can be kept in the refrigerator for a number of days.

If you need some stock, but none is on hand, chop up about 1 lb of whatever vegetables you have on hand. Then cover with 1 quart of water, bring to a boil and allow to simmer about 45 minutes in a covered pot. Drain off the stock and discard the vegetables (all the nutritional value of the vegetables has been lost into the stock). This yields about a quart of stock.

Or, you can steam about 1 lb of vegetables in 1-1/2 cups water. This will give you edible vegetables with a cup or so of stock. Use your stocks instead of water in all of your soups.

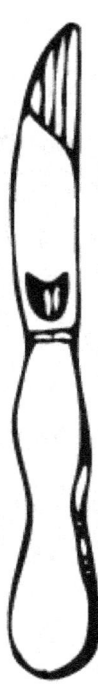

Split Pea Soup (Level I)

1 lb of split green peas (or split yellow peas, whole green or yellow peas, or any mixture of peas)
1 medium onion (chopped)
1 celery heart (chopped)
3 T Tamari or Bronner's Broth
2 to 3 cups soup stock
1 leek (chopped)
2 carrots (chopped)
½ tsp white pepper
1 bay leaf
2 tsp of dill weed
1 tsp of basil

Cook the peas as you would beans. Do not drain. As the peas cook, sauté the onion and leek in a dry pan until brown. Add 2 T olive oil, the carrots and celery heart and continue to sauté until tender. Add these to the cooked peas along with the spices. Then add soup stock to get your desired thickness…Serve hot with salad and whole grain rolls.

Black Bean Soup (Level I)

1 lb black beans
1 leek (chopped)
1 medium carrot (chopped)
2 tsp cumin
2 T Tamari
Pepper to taste
1 medium onion (chopped)
1 green pepper (chopped)
1 celery heart (chopped)
1 to 3 cups soup stock
3 T olive oil

Cook the beans; do not drain. While beans are cooking, sauté the onion and leek in 1 T olive oil. Then add 2 T olive oil, the vegetables and spices and sauté until tender. Add this to your beans when they are ready, along with as much stock as necessary for your desired thickness.

Potato Leek Soup (Level I)

2 cups cubed potatoes
1 medium onion (chopped)
1 T fresh parsley (chopped)
1 tsp white pepper
2 leeks (chopped)
2 tsp fresh dill (chopped)
2 T Tamari
Soup stock or water

Place potatoes in a pot with enough water to cover. Cover pot and bring to a boil. Leaving lid on, remove from heat and let stand 25 minutes. Meanwhile, sauté the onion and leeks in 1 T of olive oil until brown. When potatoes have steamed soft, mash into slivers with a fork. Then add the remaining spices, browned onions and leeks to the potatoes. Add more stock if you like.

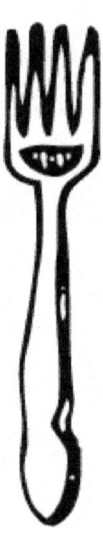

Meatless Stew (Level I)

2 cups potatoes (cubed)
2 cups carrots (cubed)
1 cup celery (chopped)
1 large onion (chopped)
1 cup cabbage (chopped)
1/4 cup Tamari
1 tsp thyme
1 tsp basil
1 tsp dill
1 bay leaf

Place vegetables into a pot or crock pot and cover with water and a lid. Bring to a boil, and then turn down heat. Add the remaining ingredients, cover and remove from heat. Allow to stand for 30 minutes. Reheat as hot as desired and serve. For a creamy stock, remove 1-2 cups of stew and blend in a blender until smooth. Return to the pot and mix well. The vegetables are best when slightly underdone. If you like, add chopped parsley, broccoli, and cauliflower. Serve hot with whole grain rolls.

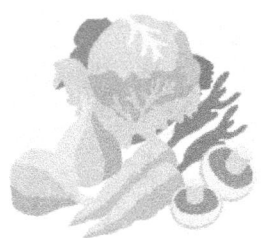

Vegetable Curry (Level II)

2 potatoes
1 cup fresh peas
2 large onions (chopped)
1 T fresh ginger root (chopped fine)
3 T olive oil
1 tsp white pepper
1 tsp tumeric
1 T vinegar
3 large carrots (chopped)
1 cup green beans (cut up)
2 cloves garlic (finely chopped)
2 green peppers (chopped coarse)
4 tsp whole wheat or rye flour
2 T Tamari
1 cup yogurt
1 cup freshly squeezed lemon juice

Dice and boil the potatoes. Steam the carrots, peas and green beans. In a dry pan, sauté the onion and garlic until brown. Then add the olive oil, green pepper and ginger and stir-fry for about 5 minutes. Then add the tumeric, Tamari, and flour. Stir in the yogurt and simmer gently until the gravy reduces by almost half. Then add the lemon juice, vinegar, white pepper, steamed veggies and potatoes; remove from heat after 5 more minutes. Serve over steamed brown rice.

Quick Pancakes (Level II)

1 cup whole wheat or rye flour
1 egg (beaten)
1 T olive oil
1 tsp baking powder
1 T honey
1 cup water
1 tsp sea salt

Mix together the flour and baking powder in a bowl. Blend the remaining ingredients in a blender and pour over the flour. Mix all well with a fork. Then cook on a hot, lightly oiled skillet. When bubbles form on the top, flip and brown side two. Serve hot with pure maple syrup.

Quick Bread (Level II)

3 cups whole wheat flour
1 cup water
3 T Brown Rice syrup
1 T baking powder
1 tsp sea salt
2 eggs

Mix thoroughly the flour, salt and baking powder. Blend the remaining ingredients in a blender and pour over the flour. Mix well with quick strokes. Place in an oiled pan and bake at 350 about 50 minutes. Top should be well browned. Serve hot right out of the pan. Or, for slices, let cool before removing from the pan, then slice and serve.

Variations: Instead of whole wheat flour, use any whole grain flour such as rye, millet, oat, barley, etc. or any combination of whole grain flours. You may have to add a dash more flour or water with these flours to get the same consistency of dough as with whole wheat flour, but the proportions given above should bake out fine.

Instead of making loaf or pan bread, form the dough into biscuit-sized rolls and place on an oiled cookie sheet. Or place the dough in oiled muffin tins 2/3 full. Bake at 350 until lightly browned on top, about 35 minutes. These rolls are so quick and easy.

You can also try adding to your dough some sunflower seeds, sesame seeds, chopped nuts, raisins, chives, caraway seeds, sliced onion, etc. or any combination of things that appeals to you. Or garnish the tops of your breads with chopped nuts or seeds.

Corn Bread (Level II)

3 cups cornmeal
2 eggs
1/4 cup honey
2 tsp baking soda
1 cup water
1/4 cup molasses
1 tsp sea salt

Mix the cornmeal, salt and baking powder in a bowl. Blend the remaining ingredients in a blender and pour over the cornmeal. Mix well and place in an oiled baking dish or square cake pan. Top with a few sesame or sunflower seeds and bake at 350 for about 30 minutes until the top is golden brown.

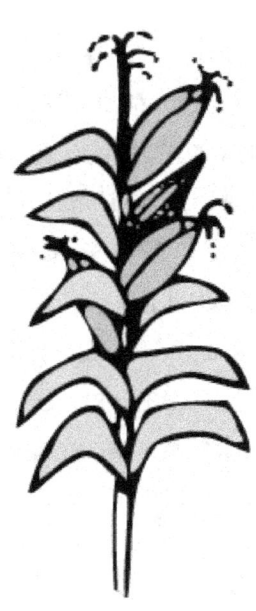

Oatmeal Bread (Level II)

1 cup whole wheat flour
2/3 cup water
2 cups leftover oatmeal
2 tsp baking powder
2 tsp sea salt
3 eggs
2 T Brown Rice syrup

In a bowl, mix together the flour, sea salt, and baking powder. Blend together the rice syrup, eggs and water in a blender and pour over the flour. Mix with a few quick strokes, then add the oatmeal and mix thoroughly. Place in oiled bread pans and bake at 350 for 50 minutes or so. Serve with honey if you like.

Whole Wheat Muffins (Level II)

The batters for muffins should be mixed just until the ingredients are moistened; over beating results in a too-dense texture. These muffins are good frozen and reheated.

1 cup wheat germ
1 tsp sea salt
2 tsps baking powder
1 tsp cinnamon (optional)
1 cup whole wheat flour
2 cups 1% low-fat milk
1/3 cup sunflower oil
1/3 cup honey
1 egg
1 T orange rind, grated (optional)

Preheat oven to 400 degrees. Into a medium bowl sift wheat germ, baking powder, sea salt, and cinnamon. Stir in whole wheat flour. In a small bowl beat milk, oil, honey, egg and orange rind together. Add to dry ingredients; mix just until moistened. Lightly oil muffin cups with vegetable oil. Fill muffin cups 2/3 full. Bake for 15 to 20 minutes. Makes 12 to 14 muffins.

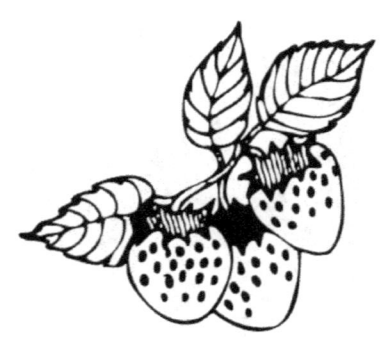

Whole Wheat Banana Bread
(Level II)

The bananas must be ripe for this dark sweet bread.
This bread keeps well and can be frozen with no loss of
flavor.

1 3/4 cups whole-wheat flour
1/4 cup wheat germ
1 tsp baking soda
1/2 tsp sea salt
1 cup ripe banana, mashed
1/3 cup honey
1/3 cup sunflower oil
2 eggs
1 tsp vanilla extract
1 cup raisons (optional)

Preheat oven to 350 degrees. In a large bowl combine flour, wheat germ, baking soda and sea salt; mix
thoroughly and make a well in the center. In a medium bowl
combine banana, honey, oil, eggs and vanilla; mix completely.
Pour into well in dry ingredients; stir just until moistened. Lightly coat a 5x9 inch loaf pan with vegetable
oil. Into the prepared pan, spoon batter. Bake for 1 hour
or until toothpick inserted in center comes out clean.
Makes 1 loaf.

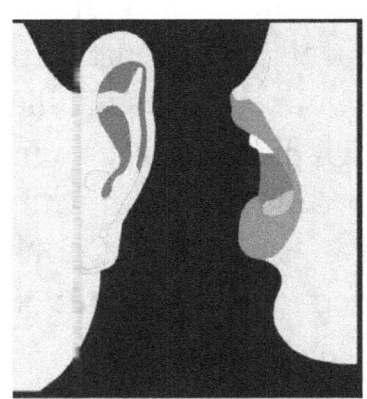

Dedication

This book is dedicated to the countless thousands of people who can and will benefit from the concepts and practices set forth within. Also to the Holy Spirit, who teaches us and guides us into all truth and wisdom concerning not only spiritual matters, but also in matters of health and physical well being. It was written for the purpose of helping any and all people who have a need and desire to make their lives and health better than they are, and who are...

WILLING TO CHANGE

whatever is necessary in order to fully achieve this goal. We also believe that this cannot be fully accomplished apart from a true experience of the love of God, and a healthy relationship with Jesus Christ as your personal Lord and Savior. "For God so loved the world that He gave his only Son so that whoever will believe in Him will not perish but have eternal life. For God did not send the Son into the world to judge the world, but that the world should be saved through Him." John 3:16-17 "For all have sinned and fall short of the glory of God, being justified as a gift by his grace through the redemption which is in Christ Jesus." Romans 4:23-24 If you do not already know Jesus, then you, too, can "Have peace with God through faith in Him. For while we were still helpless, at the right time Christ died for the ungodly." Romans 5:1&6 "If you confess with your mouth Jesus as Lord, and believe with your heart that God raised Him from the dead, you will be saved; for with the heart man believes, resulting in righteousness, and with the mouth he confesses, resulting in salvation." Romans 10:9 and 10
If you have never been born into God's family by receiving Jesus as your personal Lord and Savior, you can do that right now by simply asking Him with your heart and your mouth. Just repeat this simple prayer out loud:

Lord Jesus, I have been separated from You and the Father by my sins. I believe that You died to pay for my sins, and I choose with my heart and my mind to turn and repent from sin. Please forgive my sins, and cleanse me from them. I ask You to become the Lord of my life, fill me with the Holy Spirit, and restore me to fellowship with the Father. I thank you for saving me, and I ask You to teach me all that I need to know concerning the new life that You've just given me. I ask this in Jesus' name.

If you prayed this prayer and would like more information concerning this, you may contact us at our website, and may God bless you richly in body, soul and spirit.

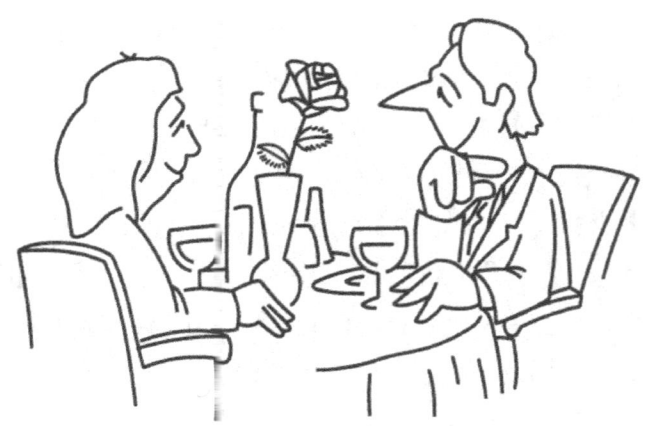

About the Author:

Kathy Stommel has studied nutrition for twenty-five years. She struggled with wanting to lose weight and look right in her teen years and got way out of balance through severe dieting. Out of great desire to change and be healthy, she began studying psychology. She then attended Lesley College in Boston and received her Bachelors of Science in Expressive Therapy. She also attended Berklee College of Music and received her Bachelors of Music.

Kathy had started her life long journey of nutrition after being told by a Medical Doctor that she needed hysterectomy because of continued severe pain. She began to read every book she could on plan, health, nutrition, and herbal healing. She went to a homeopathic MD and was advised to change her plan dramatically. She attended two-year School of Healing, majoring in Nutrition and Body Systems. She was healed of this sickness. She learned through this experience how to eat in a way that is healthy, enjoyable, and free from the bondage of obsession with food and weight.

Kathy is a Licensed Clinical Pastoral Counselor. She is a certified psychosynthesis private and group therapist. She holds her Masters from Liberty University in Lynchburg, VA. She is currently working on her PhD in Clinical Christian Counseling. Kathy and her husband are owners of Christian Counseling Associates (Christiancounselassociates.com.) She is currently working on Willing To Change II. Kathy, her husband Gary, and their three Sons; Miles, Allen and Isaiah, currently live in Nashville, TN.

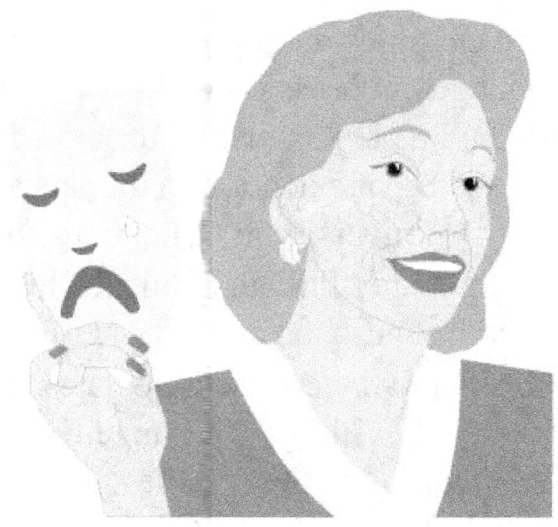

Order Reminder...

Be sure to tell your Brothers and Sisters in Christ,
friends relatives and others about the
Willing to Change eating lifestyle.

They can acquire their own copy from
www.WillingToChange.net

May God continue to guide and bless your life.

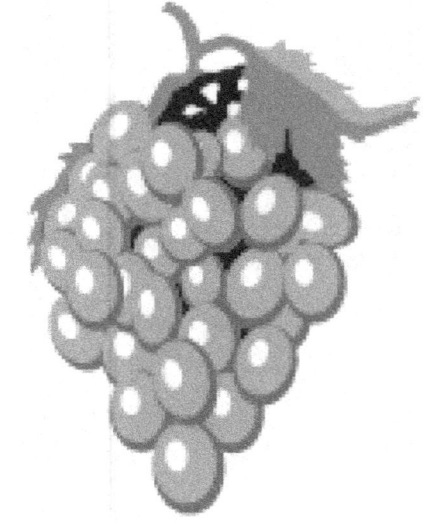

www.ingramcontent.com/pod-product-compliance
Lightning Source LLC
Chambersburg PA
CBHW081119290526
45795CB00006B/2176